Colin Rose is a graduate of Londo
of the British Association for the A
He has previously researched and
nutritional and psychological inno
scientific ground. He is co-founde
a British company now active in c
books include *Accelerated Learning* and *The Micro Diet* (with
Malcolm Nicholl).

THE MIND & BODY DIET™

Colin Rose

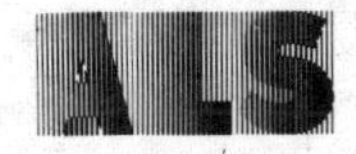

Accelerated Learning Systems Ltd

First published in Great Britain by
Accelerated Learning Systems Limited
50 Aylesbury Road, Aston Clinton, Bucks

ISBN 0-905553-29Z

Dedicated to Lena Bowles and Lena Young

Designed and typeset by
The Publications Professionals, Amersham, Bucks

Cover design by Richard Epps

Printed and bound in Great Britain by
Richard Clay Ltd, Bungay, Suffolk

CONTENTS

PROLOGUE

THE POWER OF THE MIND

Imagine you are in the kitchen. You take a fresh lemon from the fruit bowl. It is cool in your hand. The yellow dimpled skin feels smooth and waxy. It comes to a small green conical point at either end. The lemon is firm and quite heavy for its size as you look at it in the palm of your hand.

You raise the lemon to your nose. It gives off such a characteristic, unmistakable citrus smell, doesn't it? You take a sharp knife and cut the lemon in half. The two halves fall apart, the white pulpy outer skin contrasting with the drops of pale, lemon-coloured juice that gently ooze out. The lemon smell is now slightly stronger.

Now you bite deeply into the lemon and let the juice swirl around your mouth. That sharp, sour lemon flavour is unmistakable.

Stop a minute! Is your mouth watering?

It does for most people—and the implications are fascinating because, of course, nothing actually happened. Except in your imagination! Yet your mind communicated directly to your salivary glands and told them to wash away the sour taste.

The words you read or heard were not reality—but they created reality—your mouth watered.

The fact is that the subconscious mind cannot differentiate between what is real and what it believes is real. Yet your subconscious mind directly controls your actions in a very tangible way.

You have just proved something of the utmost importance. You have proved that you can deliberately direct the power of your mind to produce an immediate and measurable physical effect on your body.

Harness this power for slimming and you need never diet again.

INTRODUCTION

In the last four years, I can truthfully claim to have helped over 3 million people to slim successfully. Now I realise we were only tackling half the problem! It could have been so much better.

Let me explain.

In April 1984 I founded, together with my wife and two partners, a company called Uni-Vite Nutrition. In cooperation with a group of University Nutritionists and Doctors, we formulated a range of foods, soups and drinks that provide all of the protein, vitamins and minerals the body needs in about one quarter of the usual daily calorie intake.

Essentially, we took natural food sources such as milk, eggs and soya, removed what was surplus to requirements, such as fat, and fortified them with vitamins, minerals and trace elements to provide 100% nutrition in three of these meals a day.

The breakthrough was, and is, that the slimmer can literally live on these foods. Since the nutritional value is perfect, he or she feels well and noticeably energetic. Since the calorie level is low (normally about 600 calories a day), weight is lost at a sufficiently rapid rate to be motivating.

This simple concept of virtually fat-free food, that combines low calories with high nutrition, has been outstandingly successful.

Clinical trials proved that the foods, which taste good, could be safely used as a diet with great success. The average weight loss is 3–4 lbs a week for women, a little more for men. Moreover, these trials also showed other benefits—reductions in cholesterol levels, in blood fat level and in blood pressure.

From its start in the UK in 1984, we have successfully taken the Uni-Vite diet into all five continents and there are now Uni-Vite sister companies in Spain, Portugal, France, Holland, Australia, New Zealand, Canada and, recently, the huge US market. In all, over 3 million slimmers have successfully used the diet, without a single recorded case of any significant adverse reaction. So it's safe.

I believe that a key reason for this success and safety record is that each slimmer is treated as an individual on the Uni-Vite diet. A person's calorie and protein needs are obviously related to their size, sex, height, age and activity level. A 6 foot muscular man clearly has different protein and calorie requirements from a 5'2" sedentary woman. So different people are recommended different combinations of the food range to ensure they receive a nutritionally appropriate diet.

The result is a highly effective weight loss programme. Individual slimmers have lost 10 stone (140 lbs)—and more. Weight losses of 3–4 stone (50 lbs) are commonplace, and we estimate that more than 20 million lbs of unwanted fat have been lost on the Uni-Vite diet. That represents one and a half million stones—or, put another way, we have made the equivalent of 150,000 people disappear!!

I honestly believe it's the simplest, most effective slimming regime yet evolved, and the facts support that conclusion.

So why have I felt such a failure for the last six months?

The truth is that the track record of the slimming industry in ensuring that people **keep** the weight off is appalling.

Losing weight and keeping it off are two different problems

Here are the facts:

* Leading diet researchers Wing and Jeffries calculate that few people manage to lose more than 20 lbs on conventional diets and less than one person in ten manages to keep the weight off.

* Although the average weight loss for seriously overweight people on the Uni-Vite type of formula diet is 40 lbs, less than four people in ten maintain their weight loss for more than a year.

Put another way, the failure rate for conventional dieting is over 90%—and even for our own programme, in which I have taken so much pride, it is 60%.

I know a woman who typifies the problem. Using a variety of magazine diets she lost 8 stone. But is was actually the same one stone that she had lost eight times! And her story is all too familiar. Hardly any slimmer has escaped the frustration and disappointment of yo-yo dieting.

The truth is that most people—until now—have either failed to lose a significant amount of weight in the first place, or have failed to maintain their target weight if they do achieve it. That is despite the millions of words that have been written, and the millions of pounds, dollars, pesetas, francs, marks, etc. that have been spent.

Why?

We all got it wrong!

Mind and motivation

What's the common denominator in every diet book or magazine article you've ever read?

Calories.

Everyone tells you that you have to burn more calories than you consume in order to lose weight—and indeed, that's true. Hence the never-ending search for ever more exotic menu plans and ways to cut calories. Overlooking a blindingly simple fact.

To become slim and remain slim involves more than cutting calories. It involves motivation and mental attitude. To concentrate just on cutting calories is, at best, tackling maybe a third of the problem.

In the last six months, I have talked to hundreds of slimmers, reviewed thousands of cases and involved some of the world's leading slimming experts. As a result, I have formed some very strong and radical beliefs.

The Mind & Body Diet is the outcome. What is so exciting, however, is that it's NOT theory.

Each element has been successfully tested with people who had despaired of ever finding a solution to the problem of being overweight.

The basis

* I believe that, if you follow the Mind & Body Diet Programme, you can forget dieting as an issue in your life for ever. If you've been on umpteen diets, it's a bold promise, but it's one I know we can keep.
* I believe that losing weight and keeping it off are two different problems. Staying slim is a skill. Some people have that skill naturally—but everyone can acquire it. That's what the Mind & Body Diet Programme offers you.
* I believe that over 50% of slimming is to do with achieving the right, positive mental attitude. That doesn't happen automatically, but there are exciting new ways to make the power of your mind work for you, not against you. This book contains them.
* I believe that the need for genuine motivation has never been properly addressed. Successful slimming has little or nothing to do with will power. It has everything to do with wanting to be slim more than you want to eat unnecessarily. The Mind & Body Diet provides you with provenly successful ways of becoming and staying motivated.
* Finally, I believe that, if you have failed before, it is because "old style" dieting is psychologically virtually impossible.

As a last bit of background before we get started on the Mind & Body Diet, let me explain that last statement.

The four psychological flaws in conventional dieting

1. When you use a conventional diet, you consciously deprive your body of food.

Although your logical, conscious mind knows that you are doing this to use up the energy in your unwanted fat stores, your subconscious mind is programmed to know that, if you don't eat enough, you will not get enough nutrition, and that if you don't get enough nutrition, you'll eventually die!

Since the most basic instinct in people is the instinct for self-preservation, your conscious may say "don't eat"—your subconscious will be pleading "EAT"!

So there's a conflict, and we shall see that, when there's a conflict between the subconscious and conscious mind, your subconscious will ALWAYS win.

2. Conflict of any sort brings tension and fear. For many people, tension and fear are relieved by eating. Overeating produces fat, then they blame themselves, feel guilty and want to comfort themselves. How? By eating their favourite comfort foods!

3 Another powerful human instinct is the instinct to avoid pain and be comfortable. A person on a conventional diet denies herself or himself, and therefore feels deprived. To feel deprived is to inflict discomfort on yourself, and your subconscious will naturally resist this. The diet's restrictions are seen as a sort of punishment and, sooner or later, you rebel. In that sense, a diet can actually cause a binge!

4. Conventional dieting concentrates on the very thing you want to forget—on weight and on food. Worse still, it does so in a COMPLETELY NEGATIVE WAY.

   Conventional dieting concentrates on losing weight. It concentrates on cutting out food. It says: "Don't do this", "Don't do that". All negatives—and a mind fixed on negatives looks for failure.

Four good reasons for any past failures. Now let's look at why you will succeed this time!

THE MIND & BODY DIET PROGRAMME

This is a comprehensive programme designed to enable you to become and stay slim. There are three key elements—Mind, Body and Motivation.

1. Mind

A six-week voyage of self-discovery

The remainder of this book is split into six sections. Each section represents a week—a week in which we will explore some thought-provoking issues together and review some interesting facts about your mind and body. Many of these facts, I suspect, will be new to you. They are important, because I believe that knowledge is essential if you are to become convinced, and conviction is essential if you are to have the strong inner motivation to succeed.

In addition, you will learn how to harness the power of your mind to work for you.

All things must be mentally accomplished before they are physically accomplished. So you need to believe you will be slim, and be able to visualise yourself as slim, before you can actually become slim.

In other words, the six weeks will, as promised, teach you the skill to be slim.

Moreover, on the Mind & Body Programme your mind is fixed positively on what you will gain. It shifts you from being weight-conscious to being slim-conscious. From thinking in terms of losing weight to thinking about gaining a slim, trim body. From thinking of yourself as fat to visualising yourself as slim. All positives—and a mind fixed on positives looks for success.

Why six weeks? Because it's long enough to see major results and prove that the programme really works—but it's short enough for you to be able to commit yourself wholeheartedly.

A personalised low-calorie/high-nutrition diet

Whilst you are learning the skill to stay slim, I recommend you use the Uni-Vite low-calorie foods as the way to become slim.

There are eight basic "logical" reasons:

1. You will not be hungry—especially after the first 1–2 days.

2. You are certain of getting 100% nutrition.

3. You will lose weight quickly, which is most encouraging.

4. You begin to train your stomach to expect less bulk.

5. It is an ideal way to interrupt the very behaviour, habits and foods that have led you to put weight on.

6. You will begin to lose your taste for fatty and/or over-sweet foods.

7. You will experience the exhilaration of eating enough to satisfy you but not enough to make you feel uncomfortably full. A feeling of being in control and being aware of your body. And that is a key skill in being naturally slim.

8. The diet is inexpensive—the costs of the low-calorie/ high-nutrition foods are no more than the foods they replace.

Of the above eight reasons, I consider reasons 5 and 7 to be particularly important.

To the above "logical" reasons must be added two vital "psychological" reasons:

1. The slimming phase with the Uni-Vite food range is all positive. It emphasises eating, and because you know you'll be getting 100% nutrition, there's no conscious versus subconscious conflict. If there's no conflict, there's no tension. If there's no tension, there's no urge to eat to "feed your mind".

   This is a "Do" slimming programme, not a "Don't" slimming programme.

2. It's also a blissfully simple programme. Whereas conventional dieting often requires too many decisions and choices, the Uni-Vite programme simply promises that any three of its low-calorie/high-nutrition meals a day will provide complete nutrition in about one quarter of a normal day's calorie intake. This is why so many millions of people have already succeeded with it.

Important: I recommend the Uni-Vite diet so strongly because I believe it achieves what other diets cannot. However, I must declare an interest. I am, of course, a major shareholder in the Uni-Vite company.

To redress the balance, let me assure you that 90% of this book is about "Mind" and "Motivation", and the advice could—and should— be used in conjunction with any diet you sincerely believe will work during your weight loss plan.

Furthermore, I have included a section at the back of the book that presents you—and your doctor—with the information you need to make a reasoned decision as to whether to use the Uni-Vite diet foods to slim with and, if so, how to obtain them. For now, suffice it to say that it is a wide enough range to cater to everyone's taste.

3. Motivation

Practical support and built-in rewards

It has been amply proven that the way to success is to have a clear, written goal that is to be attained within a specific time. And to reward achievement of that goal in a positive way.

You will see that, week by week, the subject of motivation is discussed, and that your inner motivation is built up. However, we have found that a simple new idea has provided a huge amount of extra "external" motivation.

Team Trimming

There is no question that a small group of people, slimming together towards a group goal, provides a very powerful additional motivation. You reinforce each others' resolve, you give each other strength, moral support and inspiration, and the whole thing actually becomes fun!

If you are in a position to form such a group of friends, colleagues or neighbours (even 3 or 4 is enough), I urge you to apply to the address at the back of this book. We will explain how your team, and its weight-loss goals, can be registered—and how each member will be awarded a free, full-size bottle of French perfume as a reward if your team achieves its goal weight over the six-week period. (Or after-shave, if your team is male!)

In this way, you will have succeeded in combining all the motivational elements we have found to be important. You gain the very real benefits of group support, you concentrate for a defined six-week period, you have a specific and realistic goal, and you have the incentive of a reward at the end—a reward that fits in with feeling and looking good. To this I should add that there is a National Prize Draw each month for successful teams.

We have found nothing so powerful as the "Team Trimming" concept.

But what if you are not in the position to form a small team? If your circumstances make it more practical to slim as an individual?

Well, there's extra motivation for you, too.

The Advisor

Over the last five years, Uni-Vite has evolved a national network of Advisors. People who have experienced the same problems as you, but who know at first hand how well the low-calorie/high-nutrition diet works. Who can honestly say: "I've tried it and it works". Advisors have now been trained in the Mind & Body Diet Programme.

So wherever you live, you can now receive the practical one-to-one support, encouragement and motivation of an Advisor to assist you in successfully completing your own Mind & Body Diet Programme. Again, the address is at the back of this book.

This Advisor support enables you to reach for the phone instead of reaching for a sandwich!

You have now seen the comprehensive, three-part structure of the Mind & Body Diet Programme.

In the weeks ahead, you will discover that the mind unquestionably controls the body—just as the state of the body influences the mind. Dealing with one without the other cannot produce the results you want.

We will discover why it is that low-calorie/high-nutrition foods are so essential for people with a low metabolism—especially women. That's "body".

We will discover how many times you eat for reasons totally unconnected with hunger and how to reduce them. That's "mind".

We will discover why some people metabolise food so readily into fat—and how to reduce this unwanted effect. That's "body".

Mind and Body, Body and Mind. They are inextricably entwined, not just in slimming but in our whole life.

But there's yet another element. We will see how to achieve the commitment and positive attitude that assures long-term success. That's motivation.

Mind, Body and Motivation. That's what's new, and that's why this programme works.

"A sound mind in a sound body."
Juvenal

THE UNI-VITE CONSULTANT PANEL

Areas of Specialization	***Consultant***	***Country/Clinical Centre***
Nutrition	Dr B J Stordy	**Great Britain** Senior Lecturer in Nutrition, University of Surrey
Endocrinology and Metabolism	Dr Jerrold Olefsky	**U.S.A.** Professor of Medicine, University of California, San Diego
Endocrinology	Dr Juan Cabrer	**Spain** Head of Endocrinology Unit, Hospital Clinic, University of Barcelona
	Dr Galvao Teles	**Portugal** Professor of Endocrinology, University of Lisbon
Obesity	Dr M Apfelbaum	**France** Professor of Medicine, University of Paris
Cardiac Function and Exercise	Dr Alfred Wirth	**Germany** Head of State Clinic, Bad Rothenfelde, and former head of Heart Research Unit, Heidelberg University
Diabetes	Dr R S Scott	**New Zealand** Physician in Diabetes and Lipid Disorders, University of Otago
Clinical Nutrition	Dr L Levy	**Canada** Staff Physician, Hospital for Sick Children, Toronto

THE MIND & BODY DIET™

WEEK ONE

SOME BASIC TRUTHS ABOUT LEARNING THE SKILL OF BEING SLIM

1. Lapses are inevitable.

2. You can't possibly "blow" a diet in one day's lapse. At least, you can't "blow it" physically—but you can "blow it" mentally. Unless you are prepared.

   Concentrate on your ***successes***—not your failures. If you can manage successfully even for ***ONE*** day, you have the basic ability to be slim. Successful slimming—or successful weight maintenance—is purely a matter of succeeding one day at a time—and linking those days together!

3. Dieting and life are like snakes and ladders! The important thing is to make overall progress—even if it does sometimes include a slip up—or back slide!

4. You eat about 1,000 meals a year. By the time you're 35, you've eaten 35,000 meals. One good or bad meal doesn't make much difference. Equally, after 35,000 meals you won't change your habits overnight. It will take a little time!

5. Losing weight and keeping it off are not the same thing.

FIRST THE GOOD NEWS

It is a scientific fact that the great majority of overweight people:

Do ***NOT*** necessarily eat more than others

Are ***NOT*** weak willed

Do ***NOT*** have "deep" psychological problems

Moreover, it is only recently that it's "in" to be "thin". Most of the fabled beauties of history were quite well covered by our standards—Cleopatra, Nell Gwyn, Catherine the Great, Lillie Langtry.

For a woman, it is a natural part of femininity to be "curvy". For all of us, some fat stores are absolutely necessary.

So let's get our task into perspective. What we are aiming for is to be attractively slim so we are healthier, feel good and look good to ourselves.

What we are **not** trying to do is to achieve some artificial, even unnatural, standard of shape dictated by some of the fashion magazines!

Feel better?

Good! Because here comes the not-so-good news!

Whilst no one is fated to be fat, we are not all born equal when it comes to achieving and maintaining weight. Some people inherit the tendency to be fat, some people have a sluggish metabolism, and there are six biological reasons why women tend to put on weight.

So there's no need to feel guilty if you have become fat. On the other hand, the fact that there may be good reasons why you have the problem, doesn't justify staying fat. It may be harder for some people to achieve slimness, but it's never impossible. Whatever your background, whatever you weigh now, and however many times you've tried to diet before, you can be slim and remain slim. You just have to know how.

This is what the Mind & Body Diet Programme is about!

Some more good news!

We will ***NOT*** be counting calories, which I think is boring and makes food sound negative. Instead, we will become much more aware of how our body feels and will learn to trust what it wants. We will concentrate on eating the foods we really love, and we will SAVOUR them fully.

We shall also have some fun along the way!

So let's get started!

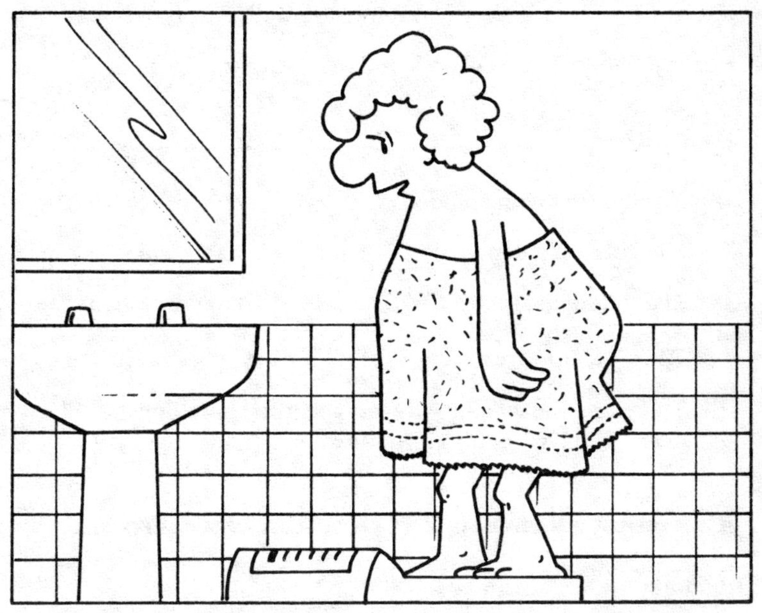

"I had no idea this towel was so heavy!"

THE MATHEMATICS OF WEIGHT LOSS

Stay with me—this is not boring. In fact, it's one of the most important sections in the Mind & Body book.

You'll see endless articles about the common sense of dieting at about 1200 calories a day. You'll also see diets printed week after week at that level.

If the first diet worked, why publish a new diet every week?

Here's the theory, the fallacy—and the facts about dieting.

The Theory

1.	The average woman needs . . .	2100 calories a day
2.	She goes on a conventional diet of . . .	1000 calories a day
3.	The difference is . . .	1100 calories a day

4. There are approximately 3500 calories in 1lb of body fat.

   Therefore, the average woman will lose approximately 1lb every $3\frac{1}{2}$ days—or about 2lbs a week.

Theoretical conclusion: *That's a nice, steady, sensible diet.*

The Fallacy

1. The latest statistics from the prestigious Dunn laboratories at Cambridge University indicate that the average woman needs only about 1850 calories a day. The result of more sedentary lifestyles, central heating, labour-saving devices, etc.

2. It's not logical to base the argument on the average woman. By definition, an average means that some women need more, some need less calories than the norm.

It is precisely the woman with a **below** average metabolism who struggles with her weight—who only has to look at a chocolate to put on a pound!

So the problem dieter may well have a metabolism some 20% lower than the average (which is now authoritatively thought to be lower than previously believed anyway!)

3. When you go on **any** calorie-restricted diet, an automatic defence reaction is triggered. Your body senses the lower calorie level and slows down its metabolism to conserve energy.

   It's an appropriate reaction for our ancestors, who were short of food, but not when you **want** to lose weight!

   This reduction in metabolic rate is about 15%.

   Although this reduction in metabolism is reversed when you stop dieting, it must be taken into consideration.

Conclusion: *Many people need a lot less calories to achieve a weight loss than was commonly thought.*

The Facts

The average woman **actually** needs . . .	1850 calories a day
The woman with a below average metabolism probably only needs . . .	1500 calories a day
Her calorie needs whilst on a diet, (after the 15% reduction in metabolic rate) may well be only . . .	1275 calories a day

Conclusion: *No wonder so many women simply can't lose weight on conventional 1200 calorie diets, become dispirited and give up.*

Even a 1000 calorie diet would, after an initial loss of largely water, only produce a fat loss of about 1 lb every 7–10 days. No one is going to tolerate that.

The above, simple calculations are at the heart of the Uni-Vite diet programme.

If you are a slow burner, the reality is that you simply will not get a fast enough weight loss to keep you motivated unless you go on a safe low-calorie diet.

Q How do you make it safe?

A Cut out the non-essential calories, but keep in the essential nutrients.

The following facts are also vital to an understanding of why the Uni-Vite diet programme is such a breakthrough.

The Facts

1. The average British diet contains almost 40% fat. It's far too high, of course, but it represents over 900 calories A DAY!
2. The average woman consumes about 10–12% of her calories as protein—about 45–50 grams.
3. The balance is carbohydrate and alcohol.
4. Even in England there is evidence of nutritional deficiency in everyday diets, and a recent University of Surrey report showed that MOST conventional calorie-restricted diets were deficient in certain key nutrients—especially folic acid, iron, calcium and zinc.

HOW THE UNI-VITE PERSONALISED DIET WORKS

Breaking the vicious circle

You have just seen why it is that so many people—women in particular—have failed to lose weight on conventional 1000–1200 calorie diets. The weight loss is simply too slow to provide enough encouragement—so they give up.

Alternatively, slimmers may be tempted by the crash diets— diets where you eat virtually nothing—or an extremely limited range of foods. You may, indeed, lose weight, but all too soon the effects of inadequate nutrition begin to be felt. You start to feel weak or unwell and again (wisely, this time) give up.

It's a vicious circle. But this vicious circle can be broken by a new generation of diet foods—foods that combine low calories with high nutrition—enabling you to lose weight at a satisfying rate, but still feel well and energetic.

The Uni-Vite range offers such foods. Each meal provides exactly one third of your recommended daily requirement of protein, vitamins and minerals—the more than 45+ nutrients the healthy body needs. So three meals provide 100% nutrition and do so in an average of about 600 calories a day, which is approximately one quarter of a usual day's calories.

There is a wide choice in the range and it enables you to eat normally. There is, for example, a nutritionally complete breakfast muesli, and a choice of nutritionally complete "Micro Soups" or "Micro Bars" that are practical for lunch. A new range, suitable for dinner, is marketed under the brand name "Whole Meals" and these, again, contain one third of the nutrients you need, but are served hot. They are filling and they include pasta-based meals, curry and chilli. In addition, there's a good choice of nutritionally complete drinks with flavours that include chocolate, strawberry, vanilla, banana, butterscotch, etc.

Not only does the breadth of choice ensure that you enjoy the meals but it enables you to "mix 'n match" the meals to ensure that you have a daily calorie level that's ideal for your personal circumstances. This, in turn, is determined by your sex, age, height and exercise level. Men, for example, need more daily protein than women and a somewwht higher calorie level. This "personalised" approach was recently endorsed by a Department of Health Report.

If you want to use this simple, successful and safe approach to losing weight **whilst** you learn the skill of being slim, you should phone or write to the address at the back of the book. You'll be advised promptly on an ideal personalised plan.

Not a very low calorie diet

The Uni-Vite foods are specially formulated to be virtually fat-free. And since about 900 calories a day of an average person's diet comes from fat, this makes the job of ensuring full nutrition in a low calorie level comparatively easy.

Low calorie level, however, does not mean a very low calorie level—over which there has been so much controversy. The UK Department of Health has defined Very Low Calorie Diets (VLCDs) as diets below 600 calories, and has recommended restricted use of these diets. The Uni-Vite Programme is therefore an ideal balance between a calorie level that is low enough to produce good motivating weight losses (about 3–4 lbs a week) but not so low as to be in the controversial area.
I believe it to be a responsible and sensible position, and one I know that most doctors agree with. Certainly, it is endorsed by Uni-Vite's eminent international medical panel.

For the reasons given in the preceding section on "The Mathematics of Weight Loss", I believe that—for the millions of people with a below-average metabolism—a safe formula diet, such as the Uni-Vite range, is the only way they can solve the competing problems of achieving a high enough nutrition level for health and safety with a low enough calorie level for weight loss.

MOTIVATION

I have tried, in this Mind & Body book, to give you all the information you could ever need to help you decide to lose weight. I will also give you several unique new methods that guarantee success in maintaining an ideal weight, if you use them.

But there's still a missing ingredient if you are to lose and maintain the weight. **Motivation.**

That's why we created the "Team Trimming" concept and the Advisor support network.

There's another kind of motivation, however, which only you can supply, because it comes from within. That's the motivation of **commitment.**

And that commitment starts with a **specific** goal. Without a clear, written goal you won't succeed. "Losing a few pounds" is too vague—it lacks genuine determination.

Setting your goal

Right now, write down how many lbs you will lose over the next 6 weeks and what your weight will be then. Then sign that commitment.

There are two big benefits to being specific about a goal. First of all, to start something without visualising your goal is like attempting a jigsaw puzzle without having the picture.

Secondly, once your goal is set, your subconscious mind will begin to accept that goal and start to figure out ways to achieve it. The mind—as you'll see over the next six weeks—is the most important part of a slimmer's body. More important, indeed, than your stomach or even your mouth!!

I am committed to losing . . . . lbs over the next 6 weeks

My weight will then be . . . .

Signed . . . .

N.B. The Table on page 199 will guide you as to a sensible weight loss depending upon your height, sex, age and exercise level. As a guide, women can lose about 17–18 lbs over the six weeks, men somewhat more—provided you've that much excess to lose!

A Motivating Graph!

Now you've set your goal, let me introduce you to a very motivational tool. A simple record of the pounds you're shedding. You'll find we've provided for the full 42 days of the programme—split into 2-day intervals. You should put a cross on the chart to show the number of lbs lost every 2 days. Then join up the x's to form a graph.

I can assure you it's very motivating to see the pounds being lost—and even if there is a period of 3 or 4 days when you are "plateau-ing", you can still see your overall progress.

This 'lbs Lost Chart' is an example of a vital principle we will be following throughout this course. The best way to **learn** is to become **aware** of your behaviour, then **review** what's happening and take **action** to correct poor habits and reinforce the good ones.

The 'lbs Lost Chart' also helps when you've got a lot of weight to lose; perhaps 4, 5 or even 6 stones. **It illustrates beautifully that even the longest journey starts with a single step.**

So, we've discussed the diet that will slim your body, and we've talked about motivation, lets now begin to examine those all-important mental attitudes.

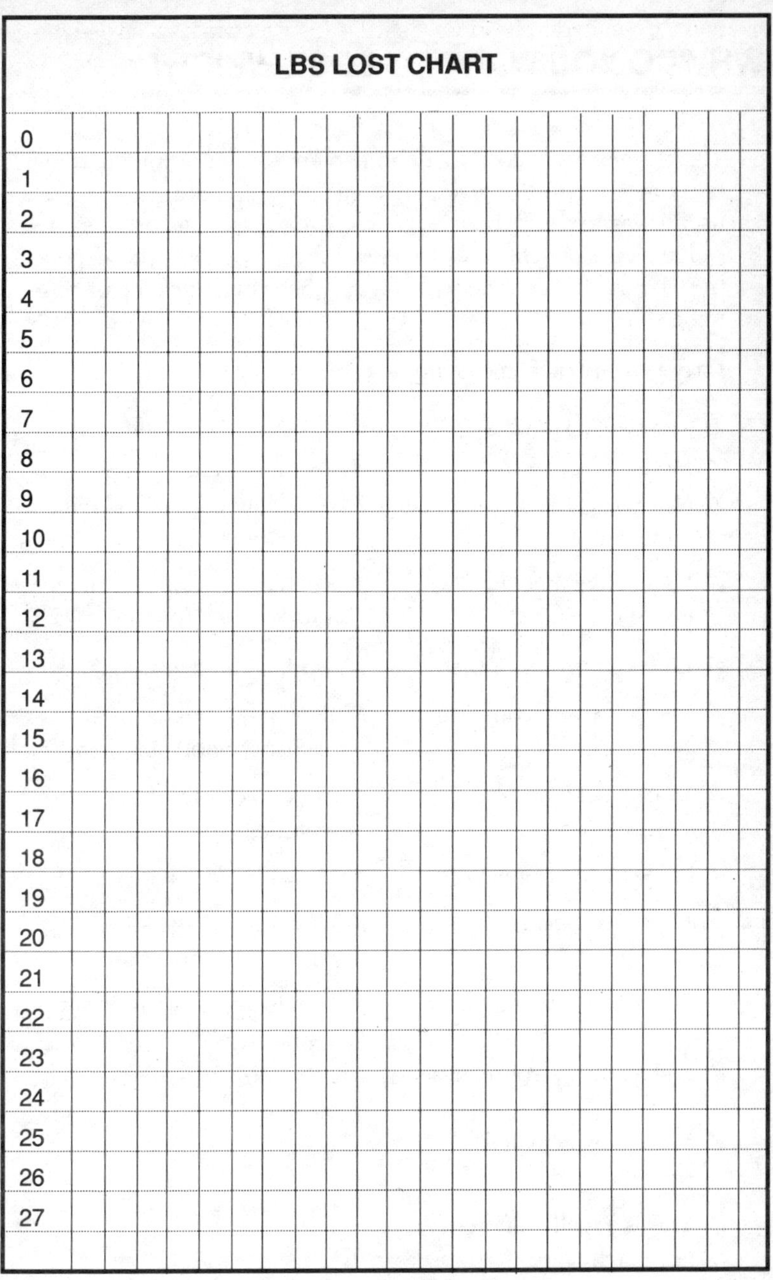
LBS LOST CHART
0
1
2
3
4
5
6
7
8
9
10
11
12
13
14
15
16
17
18
19
20
21
22
23
24
25
26
27
DAY 0 2 4 6 8 10 12 14 16 18 20 22 24 26 28 30 32 34 36 38 40 42

WHY DO YOU WANT TO LOSE WEIGHT?

There is always a "cost" to all human endeavour—either in terms of money or effort or giving up something you like. And there's a useful way to assess how ready you are to pay that cost. It's often called a cost/benefit analysis. Please list the benefits you expect from being slim and the "cost" or sacrifice you anticipate paying to be slim.

I have given you some examples:

The "benefits" of being slim

- ✓ More energy
- ✓ More attractive appearance
- ✓ I'll feel like meeting people
- ✓ Better choice of clothes
- ✓ I won't be self conscious
- ✓ I won't get breathless*
- ✓ I'll be proud of my body
- ✓ Improved health
- ✓ My doctor told me to
- ✓ I'll feel in control of myself
- ✓ Make new activities possible
- ✓ This is a really different approach

etc. etc.

The "cost" of being slim

- ✗ Feel restricted
- ✗ Having to cope with being more desirable
- ✗ Keep to the Uni-Vite diet for 4 weeks or more
- ✗ Work at the questionnaires
- ✗ Can't use being fat as an excuse for not joining in
- ✗ Need to change some attitudes
- ✗ May drink less with friends
- ✗ I'll have to make some changes in behaviour
- ✗ I'm always nervous of new ideas

etc. etc

The reason for doing this simple exercise is that you can objectively decide whether you really will pay the price. If the price is too high, you'd better wait until the benefits outweigh the sacrifices—because only then will you have the commitment. Realism is an important factor in successful slimming!

So do your benefits outweigh your cost? Only you can tell—but one thing is for sure. You will only keep the weight off if the benefits of being slim in your mind really do exceed the "cost". Your desire to be slim must be greater than your desire to eat more than you need.

If you're sure you really do want to slim, then let me ask you another question!

"As a nurse I'm naturally sceptical of diet claims, but I'm happy for you to quote my own experience and endorsement. The Uni-Vite diet works, and what's more it works where often patients had only suffered frustration and failure before."

Chris Penny, Southampton,
who slimmed 2 stone in 8 weeks

WHY DO YOU THINK YOU'RE OVERWEIGHT?

If you said: "Because I overeat", you are already prepared to acknowledge that you can influence your life and weight. Indeed, **only** you can do so!

This answer shows that you're prepared to take responsibility—and you're prepared to be objective. As you'll see, taking responsibility and being objective are two key factors in acquiring the skill of being slim.

To say that you overeat is not necessarily a term of criticism. You may well eat less than your thin friends. You may well eat less than, for example, your husband. But such comparisons are pointless. If you're overweight, you have simply eaten more than your body can burn. And that's fact, not a criticism.

Now let's see what to do if you gave a different answer. For example, to the question: "Why are you overweight?", many people answer: "Because I have a slow metabolism."

This also may well be true. Indeed, we'll discuss metabolism later in the book. But it's a fact you have to deal with, not an excuse for failing. Whether it's fair or unfair, you still need to come to terms with it.

Or again, the answer might be: "Because all my family are fat."

Again, it may well be true. The fact is that, if you have one obese parent, you have a 40% change of being overweight. With two, the odds rise to 80%.

These are indeed tough odds, but it's all the more reason for giving this six-week programme your 100% effort. It's not an excuse to fail.

The first vital point to come to terms with is this:

You are responsible.

You always have a choice of how you eat.

Fixing the blame is not fixing the problem

What do I mean by fixing the blame? Well, I mean the tendency we all have to want to blame external factors. The Government, the boss, our horoscope, our childhood, the fact that we're over-educated or under-educated, etc.

Closer to our subject, it may indeed be true that you have a low metabolism, or that you put weight on after your children. But these, bluntly, are reasons, not excuses.

I'm genuinely not being unsympathetic. I know from talking to and helping thousands of people that there are very real problems, but looking around for something—or someone—to blame doesn't get us very far. Fixing the blame is not fixing the problem.

Worse still is blaming yourself! Fixing the blame on yourself will only lead to lowering your own self-esteem, and a feeling of disappointment with yourself—and mostly that leads to over-eating!

It is curious that most people have an unrealistic expectation of themselves. They subconsciously expect perfection. yet nobody achieves 100% success. The point is to keep on improving! And accepting the responsibility for finding the solution.

Being responsible doesn't mean indulging in self-criticism. Nor does it necessarily mean you must handle it alone. That's one of the reasons we've evolved Team Trimming and the Advisor system.

A real-life example

Now let's look at a specific example of what we mean.

Scenario 1

Something happens to upset Doris. Someone at the office hurt her. She's on a diet and is grimly determined to exercise all her will power not to eat. But she's now at home, and she's angry and depressed in turns. She walks into the kitchen. She reaches for the biscuit tin. She starts to eat, leaving the tin open. She wanders around, munching and dipping into the tin.

Before she knows it, the packet is finished. Now she feels disgusted with herself—weak, worthless. She feels she can't control herself. On a scale of 1–10, her self-esteem is about minus 3!

Her next reaction is: "What the heck!" She **knew** all this weight control nonsense was beyond her, so she opens another packet and has a really good binge.

A lapse that led to a relapse, that led to a total collapse.

Scenario 2

Something also happens to upset Lara. She's at home. She, too, feels angry and depressed. She dips into the biscuit tin. Then she remembers (just in time!) the importance of being objective. She remembers (just in time!) to say: "I am responsible." She asks herself: "How can I deal with this?"

She goes for a walk to think out the problem. She comes home at least with a bit clearer mind—maybe even with a solution. And she realises she's made real progress. She didn't fix the blame: she started to fix the problem. And she didn't fall into the trap of eating as a solution.

In Scenario 1, Doris only succeeded in reinforcing her basic belief that she's a pretty useless individual. She triggered a chain reaction of negative feelings. A vicious circle—because she treated a lapse as a disaster.

In dieting, there's nothing fails like failure!

In Scenario 2, Lara broke that potential chain reaction with the simple statement: "I am responsible" and created a virtuous circle—because she treated a lapse as an opportunity to learn.

In dieting, as in life, there's nothing succeeds like success!

A final thought for Week 1

People become overweight for many complex reasons. So to become and remain slim, you must realistically expect to examine a number of issues in your life, and some of them will inevitably require some thought.

However, not everything we discuss will be exactly relevant to you, so please take a little time each week to fill in a questionnaire headed "Participation". But first, I'd like you to quickly answer some important questions under the heading "Getting Started".

I was a "professional" dieter until I tried your Uni-Vite plan, but I realised immediately it really was different. After the first few days I wasn't hungry at all and I began to feel so good. I used to be tired and lethargic all the time. Now I'm brimming with energy.

I was so ashamed of myself I used to hide behind the door whenever I had to open it. Now I love meeting people!

Bernadette Thomas, Bristol
who slimmed 4st 4 lbs in 4 months

GETTING STARTED

Fill in this opening questionnaire. Nobody will ever see it but you, but it's an important tool. Keep it and compare your answers at the end of six weeks. You'll be amazed at the changes.

Name	**Age**	**Height**	**Current weight**	**6 week goal weight**	**Ultimate goal weight**

Now answer the questions below, using the 'scale' provided. Ring the number that most nearly expresses your situation.

	Question							
1.	When did you first have a weight problem?	Age?		Reason?				
2.	When you start to eat do you usually feel:	1 Already full	2	3	4 Comfortable	5	6	7 Hungry
3.	When you stop eating are you usually:	1 Stuffed full	2	3	4 Satisfied - just right	5	6	7 Still hungry
4.	Do you eat between meals?	1 Often	2	3	4	5	6	7 Never
5.	How often are you dieting?	1 Always	2	3	4 Sometimes	5	6	7 Never
6.	How often do you eat foods you absolutely love?	1 Never	2	3	4	5	6	7 Always
7.	Do you like your body?	1 No	2	3	4	5	6	7 Yes
8.	Do you feel controlled by food	1 No	2	3	4	5	6	7 Yes
9.	Do you ever visualise yourself being slim?	1 Never	2	3	4	5	6	7 Always
10.	Do you feel guilty about eating?	1 Yes, very	2	3	4	5	6	7 No
11.	Do you eat when you're stressed or bored?	1 Often	2	3	4	5	6	7 Never
12.	Do you eat when you are worried or unhappy?	1 Often	2	3	4	5	6	7 Never
13.	How often do you have a good binge?	1 Often	2	3	4	5	6	7 Never
14.	How is your self-esteem?	1 Low	2	3	4	5	6	7 High
15.	Do you look forward to eating alone?	1 Often	2	3	4	5	6	7 Rarely

Finally, mark your own life on a 1 to 7 scale (1 meaning poor, 7 meaning excellent) for the following factors. Again, only you will ever see it, but be honest. Learning about yourself is the first step to learning the skill to be slim. And whilst the six weeks' sessions ahead won't change your job, your partner or your finances, they **will** improve your skill in living, in ways that will surprise you!

I rate these areas of my life as follows, on a 1–7 scale.
(1 would be low, 7 would be excellent).

Job satisfaction	1	2	3	4	5	6	7
Exercise level	1	2	3	4	5	6	7
Energy level	1	2	3	4	5	6	7
Family relationships	1	2	3	4	5	6	7
Health	1	2	3	4	5	6	7
Sex life	1	2	3	4	5	6	7
Stress (1 high/7 low)	1	2	3	4	5	6	7
Friendships	1	2	3	4	5	6	7

PARTICIPATION

What I learned this week

What I agreed with

Things I disagree with. Why?

N.B. Don't spectate—participate. Remember, the skill of being slim has nothing to do with will power—but everything to do with motivation.

THE MIND & BODY DIET™

WEEK TWO

WHAT DO YOU THINK ABOUT YOUR BODY?

Think back to when you really looked at yourself in a full-length mirror. Now observe your body in your mind's eye. **Don't judge, observe.** Pretend you're watching yourself on TV. Now comment on what you see.

You know something? The people who made the most positive observations about their body will have a head start in learning the skill to be slim.

The truth is that, the higher your self-esteem, the easier it is to slim.

If you hate your body, what's the reaction you feel? Disgust? Guilt? Unhappiness? And what's a typical response when you feel unhappy, or guilty, or stressed?

You eat!

And what happens when you eat? As often as not, you feel: "Oh heck, I've blown it. I might as well have a really good binge."

Does that ring any bells? It's a vicious circle! And it starts with disliking your body.

You won't find it easy to slim until you can be objective about your body. Like it for what it will become, and **start visualising what it will look like when it's slim.**

Valuing yourself and feeling good about yourself is a real secret of success. If you don't value something, you don't take care of it. If you don't take care of it, it deteriorates

On the other hand, once you start to enjoy and respect youself, to value yourself and your body, you'll start asking another very important and relevant question. Do I **really** want to eat this? Will it do me good? Do I **need** it?

IMAGINATION IS STRONGER THAN WILL POWER!

At the beginning of this book we experienced a convincing demonstration of the power of imagination, when just the thought of lemon juice triggered a very real physical reaction

Let me now demonstrate that imagination is stronger than will power.

Close your eyes. Now think hard of your front door. Concentrate so you can see it clearly in your mind's eye. Got it?

Now visualise a big, fluffy, friendly white rabbit—a rabbit as big as a large dog—sitting in front of your front door!

Now think of your front door **without** thinking of a big white rabbit.

Try harder—force yourself to visualise your front door without thinking about a big white rabbit. **Will** yourself to ignore the idea or image or thought of a big white rabbit.

Most people can't do it, for the simple reason that, once the idea of a big white rabbit is in your mind, will power won't shift it. **Because imagination is stronger than will power.**

You can only truly be in **real** control of your actions when your subconscious and conscious mind want the same thing. Or, put another way, when your "inner" self and your "outer" self want the same thing.

This idea that we have two selves, often at cross purposes, is literally true. Thus you can say you want to lose weight, yet your inner self may be resisting it strongly. And the inner self always wins!

The outer self professes to exercise will power—the inner self just goes on doing what you really want.

When you say: "I want to lose weight, but I can't give up my late night snack", it's as though there are two "yous"—the "you" that says you want to be slim and the "you" that prefers to have the snack. And we assume the problem is that the first "you " is not trying hard enough.

In fact, there's no real conflict at all. The real you is the inner you and the inner you has decided that the snack is preferable! We **all** do what we really most want—what our inner selves wish for. And mostly our inner selves want to maintain things as they are.

The only real way to succeed in slimming is to understand this and to ensure that the inner you and the outer you genuinely want the same thing. Then it's easy, because there's no conflict.

There are two keys to harmonising the two "yous".

The first is to accept the responsibility that you can indeed lose weight quickly and safely using a low-calorie/high-nutrition plan. And you can, indeed, with a moderate change in your lifestyle, keep the weight off for ever..

The second is to get **directly** in touch with your inner self through your imagination. Because imagination, as Napoleon said, and as you've seen, is stronger than will power. Your imagination can make you slim, because it will ensure that you want to slim more than you want to eat unnecessarily.

A slim "mind" creates a slim body.

The subconscious is remarkably literal. It will accept what you tell it.

If you think of yourself, and talk about yourself, as a fat person, **your subconscious will do everything to bring about that reality.** A fat head, in the sense of someone who thinks of herself or himself as fat, will create a fat body. If you think you're fat, you'll act the way fat people do—i.e. eat too much. Result? You'll become fat!

In contrast, if you think of yourself as a slim person, and act as a slim person, your subconscious will find ways to bring that about, too.

An excellent way to reach your subconscious is to use a deceptively simple idea developed by a French psychologist called Emile Coué. He taught people to make simple "affirmations". These affirmations simply consisted of positive statements, repeated frequently. In our case, you must say: "I am a naturally slim person and this whole programme is working for me". Using the present tense is important.

That's all! In these exact words. You repeat it 10 times when you wake up, 10 times during the day and 10 times just before you go to sleep.

Now, like so many simple things that **work**, it's all too easy to dismiss affirmations as simplistic and childish. Please trust me. They really do work—and here's the reason.

The subconscious mind can only hold one thought at a time and it will always accept the stronger of two competing thoughts. By constantly repeating your **positive** affirmations, they will replace any negative image you may have of yourself.

The result is that there will then be no conflict between your inner beliefs about yourself and your outer expressed intentions. Your two "selfs" will be at one—wanting the same thing.

Many people find these affirmations, these simple positive statements, so powerful that they record them onto a tape recorder and play them at home or in the car.

Affirmations are merely statements of belief. The Lord's Prayer is an affirmation. So is the Boy Scout or Girl Guide code. So are most proverbs.

Don't worry if your conscious mind doesn't even fully believe your affirmations at first! Your subconscious will begin to believe them and gradually your whole mind will come to believe them.

After all, your conscious mind didn't really believe there was a real lemon when you did the exercise at the beginning of the book—yet the subconscious suggestion was powerful enough to trigger your mouth watering—an event which most of us think of as an "involuntary action".

WHICH IS THE REAL YOU?

What you say

We've discovered that there are two "yous": the "inner" you and the "outer" you. And they don't always agree.

Please answer the following two questions:

Question 1

When you first heard about the Mind & Body Diet, how did you express your reaction?

"Good idea—I'll give it a try."

Yes? Or did you say it some other way?

Question 2

How do you normally talk about losing weight? Do you say:

"I wish I could lose weight."

Or do you express it another way?

The answers to the questions are revealing. Because we don't always mean what we say!

What you mean!

When you say "I'll try", what you really mean is: "I may fail and I'm warning you in advance that I only ever promised to try!"

Promising to "try" is not a commitment—it's an advance let-out clause! You either do it, or you don't do it. You can't "try" to pick up a pen. You either do it—or you don't do it.

Let's agree now—we're not "trying", we're slimming. No ifs, no maybes, no buts.

When you say "I wish", you're really saying: "I'd like to do it, but I doubt if I'll have the determination or ability."

A wish is not a goal. A wish is basically a vague hope with insufficient energy behind it.

The proper answer is:

"I'm committed to this Mind & Body programme. It's logical, it's proven and it'll give me a good personal insight into how to succeed. I'm going to give it time and energy because I deserve to succeed."

> *"Whatever you can do, or dream you can, begin it: Boldness has genius, power and magic in it."*
> Goethe

DARE TO TELL THE TRUTH!

How courageous are you? Courageous enough to own up, like me—**and every single slimmer in history**—to the fact that you were full of frailty? Courageous eough to answer a question honestly?

Here's the questio:.

"What have you done to put on weight, that you don't want any-one else to know?"

The answers are usually hilarious—but I'll bet you learn a lot. It may be tip-toeing downstairs in the middle of the night to raid the fridge, or that bar of chocolate hidden in your briefcase or handbag right now, that no one knows about!

There's a reason I asked you the question, and it's part of a theme I feel is important. Making mistakes is irrelevant. Lapses are irrele-vant. The only thing that matters is to be aware of our behaviour, to be honest about ourselves and learn from our mistakes (and frailties!)

What's your "dreadful" secret?

MOTIVATION

Success in dieting is like success in life. It can be summed up in one simple question:

Are you
PARTICIPATING
or are you
SPECTATING?

Participating means fully joining in the spirit of these six weeks together. Answering the questionnaires, really thinking about the issues and taking action. It means, in other words, **COMMITMENT**. Are you really prepared to make that commitment?

Here's a test of your commitment. Each week, I'm going to ask you to rate yourself as to how well you participated the previous week. The scale will be 1–10.

10 would be total commitment.
1 would be that you virtually ignored all the advice!

You should be looking for a 7 to 10 participation level all the time. That's participating, not spectating!

Who will succeed on this Programme?

I'm delighted to say that we have learned that some things are irrelevant in predicting success in dieting.

Age, for example. Older people succeed just as well as younger people.

Intelligence is another irrelevant factor. So is education. So is occupation.

So the good news is that what you need to succeed is entirely within your control. It's called commitment!

MOTTO: Don't watch your weight—watch your motivation!

THE VITAL IMPORTANCE OF SELF-AWARENESS

1–5 Eating

One of the most important ways you can gain the full control to maintain your weight is through what I call "listening to your body".

Too often we eat just because it's one o'clock, or because we passed a baker's shop, or because the children are home from school, or for any one of dozens of reasons, few of which have to do with hunger.

If you observe those maddening people—the ones who **seem** to eat whatever they want—you'll actually see that they eat in a very specific way. They certainly eat what they want, but they eat when they **really** need to—not for other reasons.

We've developed a really easy but remarkably effective idea that helps you become aware of when to eat—and when not to bother.

For fun, I've called it the Hunger-Meter. It's amusing, but it highlights a serious point—and it definitely works!

Before I explain it, please hold up your hand and make a fist. Look at it. Do you realise that your stomach is no bigger than your fist?! It's an image I'd urge you to retain—because the truth is that we actually don't need as much food as we think we do!

Anyway, back to the Hunger-Meter. Think of your stomach as a fuel tank—and think of an imaginary fuel gauge on it. A gauge that uses a 0–10 scale.

0 is absolutely empty. You're really hungry and ready to eat. 1 would be ready to eat, 2 would be at the level of "fancying something" but not desperate, and so on.

The critical point on the fuel gauge is 5. A 5 would be that lightly satisfied, comfortable feeling where you know you've had just enough. You feel really good when you get up from eating and you've got the energy to keep going.

We can guarantee you'll feel that about any Uni-Vite meal. They are all maximum nutrition in minimised calories—which is one of the reasons that people feel so energetic on the programme.

If you start eating when you're at 1 and you stop eating at 5, you'll never ever put weight on again.

We call it 1–5 eating. It means that you are genuinely aware of your body's needs and that you are **really** listening to your body.

But the fuel gauge goes higher! In fact, it goes all the way to 10. 10 is that groaning "stuffed full" feeling where you have to loosen your belt, undo the top of your skirt, and lever yourself up off the dinner table!

Don't worry—we've all felt it. But the truth is that, if you finish eating at between 6 and 10, you will be putting weight back on.

The Hunger-Meter idea is deceptively simple—but it works. If you stick to 1–5 eating, avoid the 6–10 zone, you'll never have a weight problem again.

Incorporate the 1–5 eating idea into **your** life.

I think the concept of 1–5 eating is important because, after a time, you'll find you automatically ask yourself: "Am I starting at 1, and am I finishing at 5?" You'll find, too, it's so much easier to visualise the way you feel when you can relate it to the idea of a scale—or the Hunger-Meter..

And don't forget the size of your clenched fist!

TRUST YOUR BODY

On the trials we conducted for the Mind & Body Programme, one lady was especially impressed. She found she was able to literally **sense** the 1–5 scale. It put her **directly** in touch with her feelings and body.

At the following week's meeting, she said how valuable it was. "I've only one question", she said. "It was a day and a half before I really felt I needed to eat. Is that normal?" The answer is "Yes".

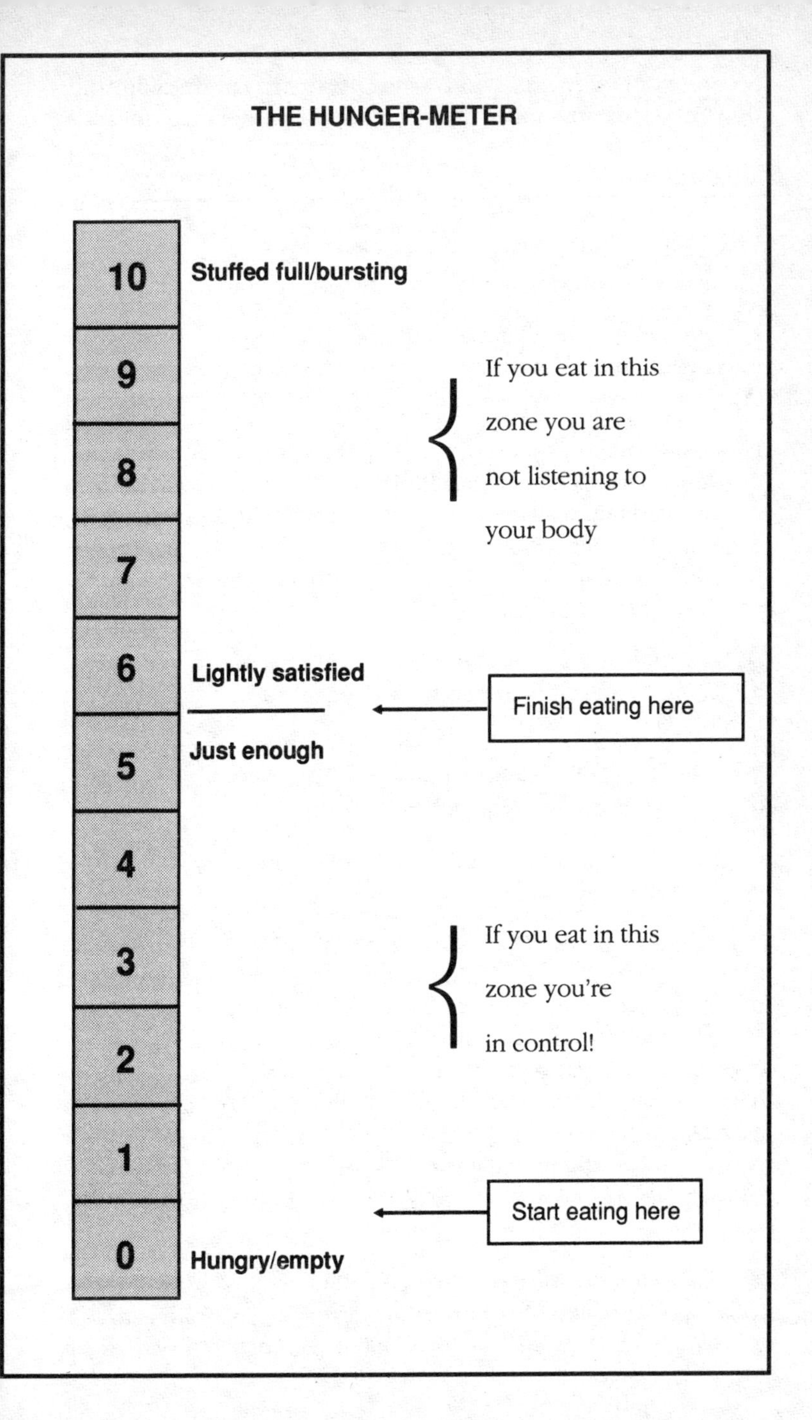
THE HUNGER-METER
10
Stuffed full/bursting
9
8
If you eat in this
zone you are
not listening to
your body
7
6
Lightly satisfied
Finish eating here
Just enough
5
4
3
If you eat in this
zone you're
in control!
2
1
Start eating here
0
Hungry/empty

So trust your body—and don't override its signals. We simply don't need to eat as much as we've been conditioned to think.

6–10 Foods

There's a second, vital aspect to the need for self-awareness, and it's the idea of making sure you **really enjoy** your food.

Now you may think that we would be encouraging you to suppress your love of food. Not so—that is the worst thing you can do!

Food is wonderful—moreover, it's vital for our very survival, and our subconscious knows this! Besides, suppressing something is an absolutely **guaranteed** way of making sure it becomes an obsession! It's like trying to suppress your anger—sooner or later the dam bursts and you're far worse off than if you dealt with the resentment at the beginning.

So how to deal with your love of food? The answer is to indulge it, BUT to indulge it in a way that will enable you to stay in control.

You see, if you only ever ate the foods you really love—whatever they are—you'd never put weight back on.

Now I realise that sounds, on the face of it, like an invitation to gorge—but in practice it isn't.

Again, think of food on a scale. A scale of between 0–10. At the top of the scale are the foods you absolutely adore. They are delicious and nutritious. They taste good and do you good. Maybe a little lower down are the foods you also love (the chocolate, the ice cream) but which you know are mainly eaten for pleasure rather than for nutrition. I think it's very important to eat them too—with one qualification. You must truly SAVOUR them. You see, if you really *savour* something, you'll find you actually eat quite slowly. Eating becomes a slow, sensuous pleasure. And you eat less, not more!

Yet how often do you see someone literally wolfing down food—gobbling it fast without really tasting it? The truth is that you simply can't appreciate your food if you rush it. If you love it, take your time. You deserve it, and in turn your food deserves your full attention.

How do you make sure you really savour your food? Use the Food-o-Meter! There's a Food-o-Meter scale in this book.

Confine yourself to the foods you **really** love, and be aware of the ones that are also worthwhile in terms of nutrition. They are the 6–10 foods.

Now the "deal" you must make with yourself is this. You can have anything you want of the 6-10 foods—because you've made a **conscious** decision that you really want them. They are, to you, really worth eating. So eat them slowly and truly savour them. You'll find that naturally you more and more choose foods that are nutritious as well as being tasty, by asking yourself a question: "Is this a 9 or 10 food?" "Will it do my body good?"

By the same token, steer off the 0–4 foods—the foods you feel disgruntled about after eating them. The ones you know are a waste of calories. They just filled you up unnecessarily and were pointless calories.

If you stick to 1–5 eating and 6–10 foods, you are genuinely listening to your body.

I think these two scales are exceptionally helpful in becoming aware of yourself.

Why you MUST eat your 6–10 foods

I said just now that I believe you should eat the foods you love—so long as you really do relish them. I should have said you **must** eat them

Why?

Because you are going to eat them anyway!

Back to Doris. Her favourite is chocolate cake. She's on a conventional diet and she's been told that chocolate cake is **BANNED.**

So she settles down to watch TV. Around 8 o'clock (researchers tell us that's THE danger time) she starts thinking of chocolate cake. She can visualise it very clearly lurking in the tin in the cupboard.

So she makes do with some nice healthy celery sticks. (She read about that in a magazine article).

Back to TV.

About 8.45 pm a vision of chocolate cake comes floating across her mind. It's stronger now and she can "smell" that rich, dark, moist texture.

So she rushes into the kitchen and wolfs down a couple of crispbreads and cheese.

Back to TV. As the end captions fade on the 9 o'clock news, the urge is irresistible. Now it's a chocolate cake frenzy! One, then two pieces are bolted down. She feels guilty—then bad about herself—then that, "Oh, what the heck" feeling—and then has another piece (on top of the cheese and biscuits, of course!)

All she accomplished was a large dose of demoralisation. Mainly because she thought of her favourite food as bad—therefore, to eat it led to guilt, and we know that guilt, blame and negative feelings are at the heart of many mental difficulties over dieting (and lots of other things, too!)

So let's agree one thing now. Being guilty is *totally* counter-productive.

Don't be guilty. Treat all your behaviour as part of the process of learning.

So what should Doris do?

Either don't have the chocolate cake in the house at all **or** list it as an 8 or 9 food (i.e. worth eating because she loves it) and look forward to it as a real treat.

Plan to relish ONE piece at, say, 9 o'clock with a cup of black coffee or tea.

In other words, make sure you get every ounce of pleasure from the food. And plan your eating, then you won't lose control and you'll feel satisfied.

Far too often we get very little pleasure out of the foods we think we most crave because they are demolished in seconds, not savoured over minutes.

Moreover, such is the perversity of human nature that when you know you can eat something—you often don't bother!

A friend of mine gave up smoking entirely by saying to himself: "I can have a cigarette any time I feel like it. But I won't just now." "Now" lasted for ever.

If you learn to incorporate the low-calorie/high-nutrition foods into your weekday routine, there will always be calories "left over" to spend luxuriously on your treats.

In this way, food becomes something you control—not vice versa. Banning foods, which so many diets do, only turns them into objects of obsession!

THE FOOD-O-METER

10	Delicious and nutritious
9	A real favourite
8	Tasted great, very nutritious
7	Tasted good, does me good
6	Worthwhile
5	Satisfying
4	OK, but questionable nutrition
3	Sorry I bothered
2	Purely filling—little nutrition
1	Waste of my waist
0	Totally worthless

YOUR NEW MOTTO – SAVOUR THE FLAVOUR!

If you ever visit Japan, you are struck by how few Japanese are overweight. I think that one of the reasons for their slimness is cultural.

If a Japanese eats out at a fancy restaurant the meal will typically contain up to 10 courses. Now with our West European cultural background we'd assume you had to be carried away from the table after 10 courses! But the point is that the Japanese don't eat much of anything. Each course is exquisite, small and full of flavour. And they relish every mouthful.

So the message is to start eating like the Japanese. Cut down the quantities and concentrate on the taste instead. Quality not quantity.

SAVOUR THE FLAVOUR. Add it to the stickers I've provided to put up around your house. (They're at the back of this week's session).

By the way, the Japanese automatically do something I've read in all the diet books. To be truthful, I've read it so often I got bored with it.

They eat on small plates. It's a fact—if you eat a small, albeit delicious, portion on a large plate, it does look "lost". And psychologically you begin to feel deprived. And that's counterproductive.

So, now you know the reason, take a tip from the Orient and use smaller plates when you savour the flavour.

THE FAIRER – BUT FATTER – SEX!

This section is for women. It's written because they are not just the fairer sex but the naturally fatter sex. It's written because it's only the ostrich who seriously thinks it can bury its head in the ground and all the problems will go away!

The truth is that women have a much tougher job to control their weight than men. But—as we've said before—that's a reason, not an excuse! No one is destined to be fat.

So let's face the facts and let the truth reinforce our resolve!

Fact 1. The average women who's in good shape will have about 25% body fat. In contrast, about 15% of a fit man's body will be fat.

Fact 2**.** Women are normally smaller than men, and therefore need less overall calories anyway.

Fact 3. Girls cannot become women—in the sense of commencing menstruation—until they have at least 20% body fat. It's nature's way of ensuring they have enough fat to nourish a baby.

It's also the reason that young female athletes—ballerinas, gymnasts—can appear so childlike. Many have insufficient body fat to commence menstruation.

Fact 4. Women naturally have high estrogen and progesterone hormone levels. The hormone estrogen causes women to deposit fat in the breasts, hips, buttocks and thighs by encouraging fat to move out of the bloodstream into fat cells in those areas.

The hormone progesterone tends to make you hungry. During pregnancy a woman has high levels of both estrogen and progesterone in her body—which accounts for the tendency for her to develop a ravenous appetite and to build up fat deposits.

In contrast, the male hormone—testosterone—actually promotes muscle growth. As we have seen, a high proportion of muscle in the body means it will burn calories efficiently, and a high proportion of fat means the body will burn calories sluggishly.

So men have a natural tendency to become lean and muscular —women to become fatter.

Moreover, estrogen encourages fluid retention—which causes rings and shoes to feel tight a few days before a period commences.

Fact 5. Pregnancy encourages fat!

As we've seen, high progesterone levels stimulate hunger and thus potential over-eating.

In addition, a pregnant woman should gain at least 20lbs— maybe 30lbs—to nourish her baby properly. But (and this is unfair) any weight gain tends to make you less responsive to the effect of insulin—the hormone whose job it is to clear your blood of excess sugar.

So pregnant women tend to produce more insulin—and high insulin levels, in turn, have the effect of converting the food we eat into fat stores.

The more children you have, of course, the more times you are exposed to this process.

Fact 6. Pregnancy increases the number of fat cells.

Many researchers believe that for both men and women there are three times in their lives when the body naturally increases the number of fat cells:

1. The last few days before their birth

2. The first two years as a baby

3. The two years before puberty.

We have seen that it is important to prevent too many fat cells being created, particularly in the third period of fat cell growth, because once a fat cell is created it is there for ever. It will shrink as you slim—but it will never disappear.

Women, however, have a fourth period in which the fat cells in their bodies increase. During pregnancy.

If you put on too much weight, too fast, during pregnancy you will lay down extra fat cells.

This is NOT a reason for dieting during pregnancy, which can be **extremely** damaging for the baby. It **is** a reason to eat sensibly and restrict your weight growth to the 20–30lbs norm. If you put on a lot of weight during pregnancy it will increase the difficulty of weight maintenance later—because you will have created not just fuller fat cells, but more fat cells.

On a more cheerful note, mothers who breast-feed their babies will be pleased to know that, during this time, fat deposits are drawn from their buttocks and thighs.

Now you may be wondering why I've written this section. It is certainly not to depress you!

Think of this parallel. Imagine you are out walking and stop to ask directions of two people. One says your destination is just round the corner, the other tells you the truth, that it is three miles away. Who does you the favour?

The first person gives you false optimism and you inevitably become frustrated and disillusioned. The second person gives you a sense of proportion and realism about the journey, and makes it easier in the end.

This section is written—like the rest of the Mind & Body Diet book—because the more information you have, the easier it is to make a sound commitment. After all, you are also on a journey—a journey to permanent slimness!

If you're a woman, there are three conclusions I'd like you to draw from this section:

1. Any man who teases, criticises or makes light of your efforts to slim should be shown the section and told in no uncertain terms that he's got it comparatively easy!
2. Women do have more difficulty with their weight, which is why a foundation of high-nutrition/low-calorie foods is so important, and why you'll see that exercise is so vital.
3. You simply can't afford much eating outside the 1–5 scale. As a woman, you don't have much margin for error, which is why the

"mind" side of this book concentrates so much on cutting out unnecessary eating. Eliminate the "mood" food and stick to the "need" food.

"Most of our team had put on weight after our children. Our lives seemed to revolve around food and we'd been on umpteen diets. The Team Trimming idea is absolutely brilliant. I don't believe we could have achieved so much without the fun of the group. We all jollied and chivvied each other along. And I'll never forget the way my husband looked at me at the end and said how proud he was. That's what it's all about."

Alison Daniels, Wiltshire,
member of the test group for Team Trimming,
who slimmed 22 lbs in 42 days

THE ROLE OF FEEDBACK

You saw in Week One a classic example of how Lara was able to use what we call "feedback" to cope with an error. The essential ingredient was that she was less than 100% successful, but instead of despair she used the lapse to learn from her mistake.

How? She analysed the situation objectively and decided how to cope better next time. A good example of turning your stumbling blocks into stepping stones!

THE IMPORTANT POINT is to recognise that you will suffer lapses—it's the reaction to that lapse that's important. Two little charts demonstrate visually the difference in behaviour between Doris and Lara.

Doris sets herself up to fail by relying on will power. We can pictorialise her failure like this:

FAILURE THROUGH WILL POWER

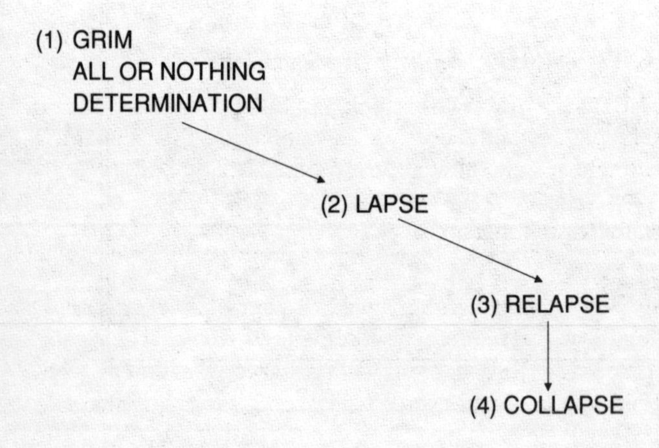

Lara's attitude was different. When a potential lapse came, she saw it as an opportunity to learn, by being aware of her actions, reviewing them objectively, deciding what to do in the future, and then taking action for the future. It's a process called feedback and this little chart shows why it works.

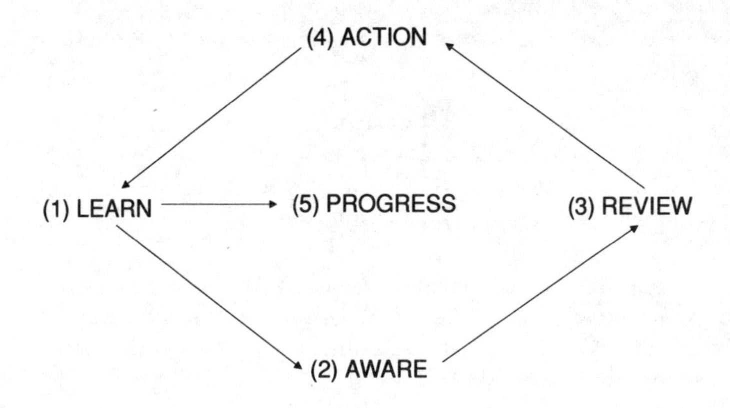

This idea of reviewing your own behaviour objectively—as if you were watching yourself on a TV screen—is a powerful help.

One excellent exercise you could do is to think over some situations in the past when you know you ate badly—or out of control. Think through what you ate, where you were and what you were feeling.

The important point is to see what patterns emerge.

You should find, when you do think it over, that there are certain times of the day, certain moods, certain situations that seem to trigger eating that's unconnected with simply being hungry.

Your own 'feedback' record

To enable you to become more aware of yourself, we STRONGLY recommend that you fill in the following feedback chart for each day next week. I realise that you will probably be eating mostly on the Uni-Vite plan—but even so the exercise is very valuable.

I appreciate that keeping these feedback records involves work, but I suggest that if your life's worth living—it's worth recording!

Moreover we've agreed that it's essential that you don't spectate—you participate. One good way of really participating is to keep this weekly feedback chart. A chart that lets you be a LARA. LARA stands for

	L earning
by being	**A ware** and
then	**R eviewing** your options
and taking	**A ction** for progress

Your personal "feedback" chart does all that. You record what you ate, your hunger scale, food scale, what you felt at the time and where you were. You also answer some specific questions—were you sitting down, were you calm, did you really savour the food? Finally, there's a space to answer whether you exercised that day.

The value of this feedback chart is that it enables you to see how to improve your lifestyle. It'll show you any consistent patterns and moods.

No one but you need ever see these records, and please remember, you're not keeping them to please anyone else— you're keeping them because the best way to stay slim for ever is to be truly aware of yourself and to take positive action to create good behaviour. And this feedback chart is the ideal way to become aware.

Finally, you'll notice there's a place to record how you rate yourself on the commitment scale!

We don't believe in counting calories—we **do** believe in keeping a record.

FEEDBACK CHART – WEEK TWO

Day	Time	Hunger Scale 1–10 Start	Finish	What I ate	Food Scale 1–10	What I felt	Sat Down	I was calm/ composed	Savoured it

My assessment of Week Two is:
(Write your suggested corrective action)

My assessment of myself on the 1—10 commitment scale is: ☐

I exercised 3 times a week for a 20 minute minimum period Yes ☐

PARTICIPATION

What I learned this week

What I agreed with

Things I disagree with. Why?

N.B. Don't spectate—participate. Fill in your Feedback Chart each week, and when you've completed it, review it and write down any conclusions you come to. Remember, the skill of being slim has nothing to do with will power—but everything to do with motivation.

THESE ARE "REMINDER" STICKERS. COPY THEM OUT AND STICK THEM ON YOUR FRIDGE, LARDER, IN THE KITCHEN!

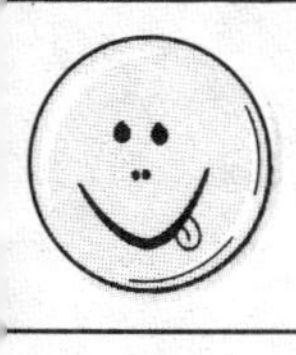

Savour The Flavour

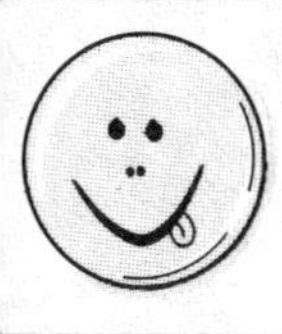

Is it a 6-10 Food?

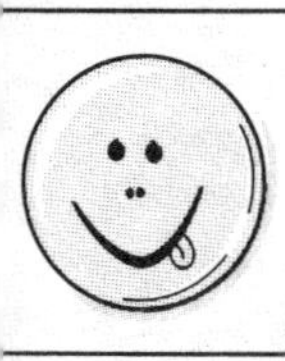

I'm a 1-5 Eater!

I'm a Calorie Trader

My Motto is "Little & Often"

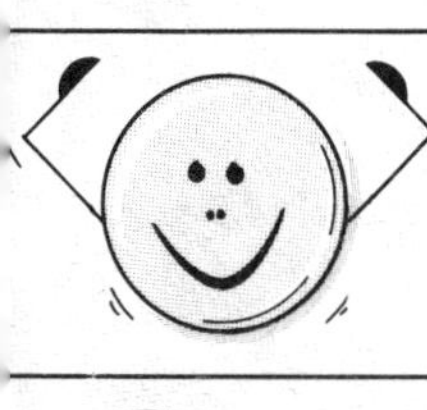

20 minutes exercise - is Not a Lifetime, but it is a Lifesaver

From Fat
I'm a Freedom Fighter!

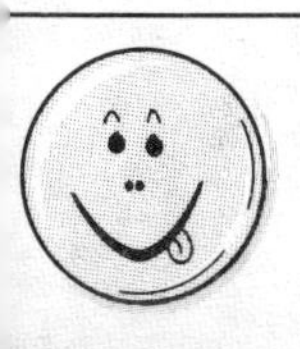

Eat to SATISFY not to FATIFY!

THE MIND & BODY DIET™

WEEK THREE

WHY DO WE EAT?

You may say: "Because I'm hungry." Unfortunately, that's normally way down the list of reasons!

You see, food works. It can work rather like a drink, or drugs, or even sex. It's satisfying—calming—a friend. The real problem is that it's also vital for our existence, so we can't deal with it by ignoring it! But we can recognise that we eat for lots of reasons unconnected with nutrition.

Food helps us through the hard times. It calms us down. It's safer than lots of other responses. It's a way to celebrate. It helps us through anger, depression, frustration. **It's easier to make a snack than make a friend!** However, as with so many friendships, it's up to us to ensure that the relationship doesn't get out of our control.

If we use food to deal with stress or anger or unhappiness, it's pretty obvious we're trying to deal with symptoms, not the real cause. In fact, if we eat because we are, for example, unhappy, we'll only end up with two problems—the original problem and an overweight body too! So it is worth tackling the real prolem.

Let's make a list together of why we eat other than the obvious reason. Think back to some past eating occasions and be honest! You'll find a lot of food is "mood" food!! In fact, a recent survey showed that 75% of overweight people ate extra because they were worried or stressed, and 95% ate more because they were tired or bored.

Reasons for eating – past occasions

Here's a check list to set you thinking—and to add to!

To make the exercise more instructive, think not only about what mood you were in but where you were and how you ate.

Here's a couple of examples to start you off:

The mood I was in	***What I ate***	***How I ate it***
Bored	Peanuts/crisps	Watching TV
Tense	Chocolate	Gulped it down
Angry		
Depressed		
Lonely		
Disgusted with myself		
Feeling insecure		
Defeated		
Elated		
Felt good		
Mind in neutral		
Envious		
Rebellious		
Feeling sexy		
Rewarding myself		

Do you begin to see common patterns?

Fatifying or satisfying?

I'd like you to think about a recent meal. A meal you remember in detail, that in your heart you know was a "fatifying" rather than a "satisfying" meal. A meal that contributed much to your waistline and little to you well-being.

What did you eat? How? Sitting? Standing? What was going on? Was it calm? Noisy? What else were you doing? Did you really savour the food? What were your feelings? Were you eating on the run, gobbling food down almost untasted, watching TV, reading a book, so you didn't even notice? Did you have the cheeseboard on the table, so you just cut at it without noticing how much you really ate?

Fatifying meals involve lots of unconscious calories. Satisfying meals are ones you enjoy, where you savour the food. Conscious calories!

What are the three most fattening things you can think of? Chips? Pork pies? Milk shakes?

The real answer is:

GUILT
LACK OF SELF-ESTEEM
STRESS

Do you agree? Do you see why? Which of your moods or situations triggers unnecessary (i.e. 6–10) eating?

The following is a very personal exercise and I hope we've come far enough for you to trust me when I say it may be important for you. Equally, it is possible that it will not be relevant to you—if so, read it, acknowledge the common sense behind it, and pass on.

The basis is that sometimes, for some people, their overweight started with a specific event, or incidents, in their lives. Events with a high emotional content.

The sort of event I have in mind would be:

> leaving home, a love affair, marriage, getting pregnant, having children, a new job, the failure of the marriage of someone close to you, a bereavement, losing a relationship.

Sometimes the events are happy, sometimes they trigger negative feelings.

How do you know if there is an emotional content to your weight problem? If negative feelings might still be influencing your weight? Go over in your mind the most important, or the two most important, events in your life. Think over where you were, what happened, who was there. Now think whether your weight changed as a result.

If it did, there's something important for you to do—something that could be a key to learning to be naturally slim.

It is to appreciate that what is past really is past. That it can have no direct relevance today.

One of the wisest thoughts I ever heard was that forgiving others is a wonderfully selfish thing to do—because the only peson it benefits is you!

Think about it. Forgiveness enables you to let go of the resentment and anger that can impoverish so many lives. Resentment and anger are negative thoughts and negative thoughts lead to low moods and low moods lead to eating in compensation! And com- pensation eating leads to feelings of failure, which leads to even more eating! Another major vicious circle!

If forgiving others is wonderfully selfish and essential, forgiving yourself is even more important!

If at any stage in the past you've felt a failure, it can be a dreadfully self-fulfilling prophecy. Your subconscious is constantly looking out for proof. So you concentrate, for example, on all the times you lapsed on a previous diet—forgetting the days you succeeded.

I'm sure you've heard of *The Power of Positive Thinking*—written, in fact, by Norman Vincent Peale. It's an inspiring book. Yet too many people subconsciously write their own opposite version—*The Power of Negative Thinking*. Unfortunately, it's every bit as influential. But you can break through such a vicious circle once and for all.

You can break through that vicious circle by:

a. Recognising that whatever is past is really past—that you can observe the past, and acknowledge it, without letting it control you. Indeed, the very act of recognising and acknowledging a past cause is more than half way to the solution. Think of any past failure as a sack on your back—and delight in metaphorically shrugging it off.

b. Resolving to live in the present—concentrating on your successes and building on them. The philosopher, Bertrand Russell, put it ideally:"Every day is a new life to a wise man."

c. Feeling good about yourself. These six weeks are designed to give you a new insight and strength. Feeling good about yourself is about the most important thing you can do to be slim.

MOTIVATION

The opposite of motivation is demotivation, and the most demotivating experience is failure. The most certain way to fail is to set up an all-or-nothing approach to your diet.

Here's the way to **guarantee** failure! Grit your teeth and say:

"I'll **never** have a McDonalds Milk Shake again."

"I'll **always** control my urge for chocolate in future."

"I'll have a salad **every** lunchtime."

"I'll cut out bacon and eggs **entirely** and just have a Uni-Vite Micro Muesli every day."

The fallacy of all these statements is that the thinking is black or white. Good or bad. The sort of "all or nothing" thinking that says that "chocolate's a bad food". Right? Wrong! The bad thing is **excess** chocolate. Unnecessary eating.

The alternative to this type of false will power is control. Saying: "I shall have some chocolate, but only enough to satisfy my taste, not threaten my waist." Will power only comes to equate to denial and feeling deprived—and always ends in a "frenzy" when the dam bursts!

Instead, recognise that no human endeavour is 100% perfect. The point is to make progress and learn from our mistakes, not wallow in self-criticism.

"Will power" is the wrong term anyway! It implies that there's a struggle going on which can be won by sheer effort and determination.

That's simply not the case. The truth is that you have to genuinely want to stay slim more than you want the piece of chocolate cake! Until the image of being, slim and the advantages of being slim, are more important to you than the (often) subconscious advantages of being fat—you won't succeed. Not because you lack will power, but because you lack a **genuine** desire to be slim in the first place.

Remember—you always have a choice, and the choice you make indicates what you really want far more accurately than what you **say** you want.

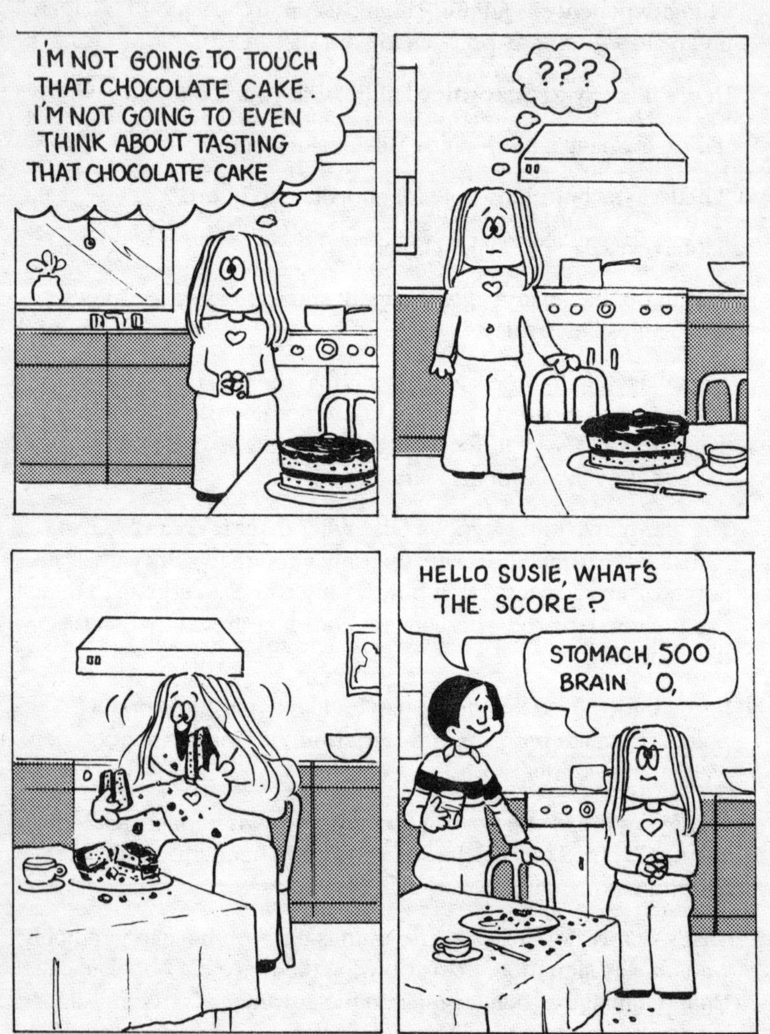

USING YOUR MIND TO MAKE BETTER CHOICES

We've found that we all eat for lots of reasons other than being hungry. If you eat on the 1–5 scale, you'll remain slim for ever—it's the 6–10 eating that makes you fat.

You can summarise the whole of this six week programme in a single sentence:

"If you stop feeding your mind and only feed your body, then you can forget dieting as an issue in your life."

Feeding the mind is eating when you're not really hungry. Eating in response to a mood, or in response to one of the eating traps we'll discuss.

But, of course, if you decide **not** to eat in response to a mood, you have to find another way of dealing with the situation. And that's what this key section is about.

As a result of this programme, we now recognise that we eat when we're not genuinely hungry—when we are:

bored, depressed, lonely, worried, tense, angry, distracted.

These are all internal triggers to unnecessary eating.

We also often eat when we're not genuinely hungry—when we:

see a TV commercial, see a magazine article, smell food, see food lying around, see a fast food sign, watch TV, etc.

These are all external triggers to unnecessary eating.

In Week Four, we look at some successful tactics to avoid a lot of this unnecessary eating.

But there's another way—a potentially much more powerful way, because it tackles the problem at its source, which is in your mind. It puts you in control of your mind, not your mind in control of you!

Let's say that, as a result of your increased awareness of your behaviour, you come to the conclusion that your main problem is eating when you're bored and down in the dumps. That's when you reach for the chocolate box.

Swish/Zoom!

So how to change? The answer is to use what we call the "zoom" technique (others call it the "swish" technique—you'll see why!).

What I can promise is that it is a fantastically powerful mental technique for changing a habit. I have seen someone who had bitten his nails for 20 years stop for ever in 10 minutes of using this method. The beauty is that anyone can do it and it's actually rather fun while you do it—but the sense of control it gives you is the real exhilaration.

Here's how you can use the zoom to control unwanted eating habits. Purely for the sake of illustration, I'm going to use the example of someone who wants to stop bingeing on chocolates.

Step 1

Start by identifying the habit or problem for which you now want a new and better reaction. Identify when and where this problem or habit occurs. In our example, it's bingeing on chocolates.

Step 2

Now imagine your eyes are a movie camera. See the situation just before you start the old habit—the one you want to kick (for example, see your hand reaching into the chocolate box and coming up towards your mouth).

Some people find it easier to get a clear image when they close their eyes. So take your time and get a really sharp picture.

Now freeze frame on that picture and put it aside for a minute.

Step 3

You now need to form a new picture—this time, of you reacting differently—the way you want. So decide what the **new** behaviour is going to be. Maybe it's putting the chocolates away. Have you decided?

This time, form a strong mental picture of yourself reacting in the new way, but see yourself in the picture—as if you were starring in the mental movie. Adjust the picture of yourself reacting in the new way so it's really clear, sharp and bright. Maybe you should turn up the sound or brightness! Do you see yourself up there **full screen**?

Take time to make a really attractive picture. Now put the new picture aside too.

Step 4

Next, bring back the first picture—the one with the old habit. Make it big so that it occupies the whole movie screen in your mind.

Step 5

Now in the lower right hand corner of the picture, put a dim, postage-stamp image of your new behaviour sequence. The new reaction you've decided on. Imagine it to be like one of those inset pictures you sometimes get on a TV screen.

Step 6

Now comes the fun bit. Here's the "swish" and the "zoom". I want you to make the current big picture—the one with the old habit in it—swish backwards fast until it reduces to nothing. At the same time, ZOOM the small picture—the one with the new behaviour —forward, making it vivid, loud and bright. Make sure it completely fills the screen, obliterating the old image.

The simultaneous swish back and zoom forward should be done really fast. In a second or less.

Two important points:

Do the whole thing with great enthusiasm and excitement (I'll tell you why in a minute).

Secondly, you MUST make sure that you blank out your mental screen completely after you have finished the swish back/zoom forward.

Step 7

Now repeat the whole process for a total of five times very quickly, but making sure you blank out the screen between each swish/zoom.

Step 8

This is the final step, and the test. Try to make the first picture again (of the old habit). If you find it's now more difficult to hold that image, and it begins to fade, you have succeeded. You have succeeded in giving your mind a new direction . . . and your behaviour will follow. You'll be surprised at the changes that can occur.

If you can still hold a strong image of the first picture you made (the old habit) then go through each step again from 1 to 6, taking time to create more vivid, powerful images to work with.

Now here's the fabulous part of what you've achieved. You can use this swish/zoom technique ANY TIME you want to change the way you react to a particular problem or situation. But use it for precise situations, not general ones.

Here's what you've done. You took a response you don't like—e.g. bingeing on chocolates when you see the box—and you've created a new automatic response to that same situation. Certainly you've done it so far only in your mind, but because your subconscious considers mental reality every bit as real as physical reality (remember the lemon!), you've created a new actual habit, too.

Now I'm fully aware that many of you will be sitting there saying: "How childish!" or even "How odd!"

Let me reassure you. Your subconscious is very literal and is very childish. You don't reach your subconscious with logic, you reach it with emotion and excitement. That's why doing the swish/zoom with enthusiasm and excitement is important.

The truth is that old behaviours can be changed amazingly fast with this technique. By manipulating pictures in your mind, you can create a new physical reality—just as you did with the lemon.

I used an important phrase just then: "You manipulated the pictures in your mind". Think of yourself as a movie director. If you have something to do that worries you, picture it—then push the picture backwards so that it becomes smaller and dimmer and darker. It now becomes something that literally **shrinks** in importance, and that you can cope with.

Let me give you a 100% guarantee. This mental manipuation works. It works fast and it works effectively. But you've got to throw yourself into it wholeheartedly.

Let me also make this point. I've had people who object to the idea of manipulating pictures in their own minds. Yet every belief, every habit you've picked up is itself a form of manipulation—but someone else did the manipulating! A friend, a colleague, a parent, a magazine article or TV programme influenced you subconsciously in the past to think or act a certain way. This time you, and only you, are in charge. I think the prospect of controlling my own mind in a totally positive way is extremely exciting and I hope you do too.

To repeat, if you don't do it, it can't work for you. If you **do** do it, it will give you a wonderful feeling of being in control. Because now you control your mind—it doesn't control you.

> *"There's nothing good or bad but thinking makes it so."*
> Shakespeare (Hamlet)

THE ROLE OF EXERCISE – WHY IT IS SO IMPORTANT

First a reassurance. We're not talking weight training or Jane Fonda style "no pain no gain"!! We're talking the fact that the optimum amount of exercise for you is enough physical movement to increase your heart rate for a twenty minute continuous period. There's no need to do that more than three times a week.

Three x 20 minutes is one hour! So are you prepared to give yourself one hour a week out of the 168 hours you've got? That's not the minimum you need—it's an optimum exercise programme!! And here's the really good news. Brisk walking fits the description! That's all. No pain—lots of gain! The definition of brisk walking is 3–4 miles an hour.

Here are the 10 benefits from giving 1 hour out of 168 to making your body feel good.

Most people only know the first.

1. ***Exercise burns calories.***

2. ***Exercise counteracts the effect of being overweight.***

   Exercise can help lower blood pressure and cholesterol. In fact there are two types of cholesterol—a beneficial form of cholesterol called HDL, which actually helps guard against heart disease, and a form that's associated with heart disease called LDL.

   [The HD stands for High Density and the LD for Low Density]

   So what you want is more HDL and less LDL cholesterol. That's exactly what exercise can help do for you.

3. ***Exercise preserves body muscle***

   One of the vicious circles of dieting is that it takes less calories to sustain 1 lb of human fat than 1 lb of human muscle.

And when you put on weight you gain far more fat than muscle, of course.

Worse still, if your weight yo-yos up and down you'll find that a higher proportion of your body weight becomes fat. So you can maintain the same body weight with fewer calories. Moreover, as we get older, more of our weight is fat, less is muscle.

It's no wonder that keeping your weight down needs effort!

Exercise provides a major benefit in that it increases the proportion of muscle weight to overall weight in your body. Your body looks much better—and because it has more muscle, it burns more calories! You see, muscle cells are like little furnaces busily metabolising food for energy, whereas fat storage cells are just that—mostly inert depots of fat that burn energy much more slowly.

So the more lean muscle tissue you have, the more calories you burn, and the easier it is to keep the weight off. And because a pound of muscle is smaller and more compact than a pound of fat, your body will be sleeker and shapelier and nicer to touch.

4. ***Exercise increases your metabolic rate***

Exercise will also speed up your general metabolism and the rise in metabolism can last several hours after you finish exercising. So you burn more calories.

That's important, because whilst you are on any diet, there is an inevitable slow-down in your metabolism as your body tries to conserve energy. Exercise counteracts this reaction and makes your weight loss easier and faster.

Once you've lost weight, regular exercise will also help you maintain it more easily. There is a very important reason why. Elsewhere we talk about the fact that the body seems to have a "set" point. A weight it gets accustomed to. When you lose weight there is a tendency for the body to want to adjust back to the original, higher weight.

The only mechanism for lowering the "set point"' seems to be exercise. With exercise, the body accepts the new, lower weight as "natural" and adjusts to it.

5. *Exercise helps control appetite*

It does so in two ways.

* Exercise increases the level of the hormone noradrenaline in your blood up to five times normal level. [Pronounced NOR-A-DREN-A-LIN] It can also increase adrenaline levels by 2–3 times.

  Why is that good? Well, noradrenaline inhibits your hunger and raises your metabolic rate—the rate at which you burn calories. Its chemical cousin, adrenaline, does the same.

  Moreover, adrenaline is a powerful mobiliser of fat from out of the fat cells and into the blood to be burnt. And that's what you want!

* Exercise increases your production of a chemical called serotonin. When this chemical reaches the brain in high levels, it switches off your hunger.

  In addition, regular exercise releases natural chemicals in the brain called opiates—and these make you feel happy.

6. *Exercise makes you more alert*

As you exercise, your breathing gets deeper and more oxygen reaches the brain. So you react faster and you become more alert and creative. The Greeks knew this, and used to encourage their Senators to walk around whilst debating politics.

7. *Exercise provides self-confidence*

People who exercise have the best chance of achieving and keeping to their target weight. Not just because of the calories burned or metabolic boost—but because they are committed, and feel they are achieving something worthwhile.

8. *Our bodies were designed for exercise*

We evolved from ancestors who had to move to survive!

As little as 60 years ago, most people earned their living by the "sweat of their brows"—by manual labour.

Evolution didn't design our bodies to sit in cars, ride in lifts and loll around watching TV! (Nor did evolution reckon on the calorie-packed processed foods that dominate our diets these days.)

So getting out for a brisk walk three times a week isn't really any more than you need to do. Not only will it reduce stress and improve digestion and make weight maintenance much easier, but it gives you a whole feeling of alert well-being. Most experts also agree it can add years to your life!

If someone launched a product with all those benefits it would become an overnight best-seller!!

The reason I recommend walking, at least to start with, is that:

—anyone can do it

—it's enjoyable

—it's free

—it can be social

—**and** (*the clincher!*) walking one mile burns almost as many calories as running one mile! Of course, running for 10 minutes burns more than walking for 10 minutes, but since you'll spend longer walking the same distance as running, the calorie burn is pretty much the same.

So never miss an opportunity to walk. Deliberately take the stairs, not the escalator. Walk to the shops, don't drive. Make it part of your lifestyle.

And if you do decide to do any other exercise, make sure it's one you enjoy—otherwise you won't keep it up.

Finally, you should be aware that the key to conditioning exercise is continuity. Although playing tennis, for example, is enjoyable, it is inevitably stop/start. The sort of exercise that does you the most good is the type that increases your intake of oxygen and raises your heartbeat for a 20 minute continuous period, but without making you breathless. You should be able to exercise and talk at the same time.

So you do not need to be a sportsperson to get the benefit.

9. Inactivity is stressful

Surprising but true. Inactivity reduces our hormone output and tiredness becomes a way of life. So we feel stressed! Not only does stress, for example, use up the Vitamin C in our bodies faster than normal (as does smoking), but if you're stressed, what do you do?

Eat!

It's all another vicious circle. Exercise breaks it by stimulating a whole series of hormonal and chemical changes in your body that reduce your desire to eat, increase your metabolism and drive fat out of your fat stores. That's all in addition to the direct calories you burn.

10. Exercise makes slimming much easier

Dieting advice traditionally concentrates on cutting intake of calories. However, increasing calorie expenditure—in the form of exercise—works just as well. And the combination of the two, i.e. cutting down on unnecessary calories and simultaneously boosting the number of calories you burn, is the ideal.

In fact, I would go as far as to say that, if you follow a lifestyle that does not do both, you are making it unnecessarily tough on yourself. Dieting without exercise is like fighting the flab with one hand strapped behind your back. It's a recipe for yo-yo dieting.

Action

Write down all the advantages of exercises that you can remember. There should be at least 12!

Make a resolution in writing to commence an exercise programme today.

Are you participating—or spectating?

This week we've discussed lots of important points, including two of the most important actions you can possibly take—an exercise

I'm fully aware that the zoom technique will appear unfamiliar —even strange. However, I know it to be very, very powerful.

If you don't use it, you are effectively saying that you are content for previous experiences, past (often random) events and other people to shape your attitudes and beliefs, rather than for you to deliberately shape them yourself.

Do try it.

And if you don't exercise, you are passing up the certain chance to boost your metabolism. It's **got** to be worth it!

"My weight loss on Uni-Vite saved me from having to undergo a back operation. I have never felt better in my life - nor looked it."

Jill Saville, Lincoln,
who slimmed 3 st 7 lbs in 11 weeks

FEEDBACK CHART – WEEK THREE

Day	Time	Hunger Scale 1–10 Start	Finish	What I ate	Food Scale 1–10	What I felt	Sat Down	I was calm/ composed	Savoured it

My assessment of Week Three is:
(Write your suggested corrective action)

My assessment of myself on the
1—10 commitment scale is:

I exercised 3 times a week for a
20 minute minimum period Yes

PARTICIPATION

What I learned this week

What I agreed with

Things I disagree with. Why?

N.B. Don't spectate—participate. Fill in your Feedback Chart each week, and when you've completed it, review it and write down any conclusions you come to. Remember, the skill of being slim has nothing to do with will power—but everything to do with motivation.

THE MIND & BODY DIET™

WEEK FOUR

IS YOUR PROBLEM A FAT HEAD RATHER THAN A FAT BODY?

We're creatures of habit and we're far more psychological beings than physical beings. We carry around with us beliefs about food, weight, eating, etc. that hold us back from being the trim, slim person that we know we can be, and deserve to be. They are the beliefs of a "fat head"—and a fat head leads to a fat body!

You should take 3–4 minutes to list your beliefs about food. When you've made your list, you'll see plenty of beliefs that simply don't square with 1–5 eating, 6–10 foods and the control you're developing from your feedback records.

I've made some comments on some typical beliefs that all too commonly hold us back:

Some typical "fat headed" beliefs	***Comments***
I need 3 square meals a day.	Maybe not—if you're eating 1–5.
I always gain weight on holiday	Not necessarily—if you eat 1–5 and 6–10 foods
Fat people are jolly	Really? Then why do so many people feel depressed about their weight?
If I eat one crisp/peanut I'll eat the lot	Not if you stop at 5 . . .
If you're fat as a child, you'll be fat as an adult	That's an increased probability, not an excuse
If I paid for it, I'm going to eat it up	Why pay to be fat?
I ***have*** *to clean my plate.*	Why? That goes back to the days of food rationing! Stop at 5.

It's impolite to refuse any food	It's not impolite to ask for portions you'll savour while you're out. It's a compliment to say "I want just enough so I'll really enjoy it."
The faster you lose weight, the faster you'll gain it back	No basis in fact. The only thing that matters is learning to adjust.
If you don't eat less when you've lost weight, you'll put it all on again	True—but if you listen to your body you won't **want** as much.
Losing weight makes me look scraggy	A pure excuse. On the Uni-Vite programme your skin remains taut and glowing.
If I skip meals, I'll feel dizzy or weak	If you've got your basic nutrition, you'll be fine.
I'm addicted to chocolate	You're only addicted to trying to solve "mood" with food. If you love chocolate, savour it—don't scoff it.

WHAT YOU 'SEE' IS WHAT YOU GET!

We've just looked at ways in which our "beliefs" about food can put obstacles in the way of permanent slimness.

This problem, however, pales into insignificance when we look at the effect that our image of ourselves has on our behaviour.

The truth is that you will never be physically slim until the image you have of yourself is of a slim person.

Fortunately, it's not difficult to achieve that, once you know how.

There is a remarkable technique, now used by all the top sports stars, called "imaging". They are taught to visualise themselves hitting a perfect golf shot or tennis shot.

They literally "see" the ball in their mind's eye, feel the perfect connection, see the club or racket hit the ball, see the trajectory of the ball. It's called "Inner Golf" or "Inner Tennis". Other sports stars use it too—for "Inner Skiing", for example. You can use it for "Inner Slimming".

Inner slimming – or the power of visualisation

To bring to bear the power of your mind, you merely need to "image" yourself as slim, happy and confident in your mind's eye. It's the process of taking your affirmation and creating a picture with it—an image of your ultimate goal. An image of you confidently and instinctively eating nutritious, delicious foods on a 1–5 hunger scale. An image of you in the sort of dress, suit, swimming costume you always wanted to wear. An image of you at peace with yourself.

I recently read a book about the 100 most successful people of the 20th century. There was not a single one of these successes from all walks of life who did not use the power of visualisation —visualising their goals. You must do the same.

Projecting your goals clearly and vividly on the "TV screen of your mind" is one of the fundamental secrets of success. And nowhere is it more important than in attaining and maintaining your ideal figure. Especially since it's not dieting that's the objective—it's a healthier, more attractive, more energetic you!

So sit quietly and form a strong mental picture on that "inner TV screen". See yourself at your target weight. Feel the sleekness of your body. Hear the complimentary comments of those who love you. See how you walk, move. Feel it in detail. Imagine you have controls so that you can make the picture sharper, brighter, more colourful.

The key to "inner slimming" is repetition. You MUST keep repeating this private "video sequence" day after day. Do it for 20 times every day and you'll have the most powerful ally possible—your subconscious mind!

The truth is that, unless you change your body **image** from fat to slim, you'll never make a permanent change in your physical body from fat to slim.

Remember the lemon! Your subconscious cannot differentiate physical reality from "mental" reality.

Create the mental reality of a slim body and your mind will find ways to create the physical reality of a slim body.

The mind rules the body

Let's summarize some important points we've learnt so far about the mind..

* What you say, and what you really mean, are not necessarily the same!

* Unless your "inner" beliefs and subconscious objectives match your "outer" goals, you will always struggle. Your "outer" statements we think of as will power, but that will always be overruled by your subconscious beliefs and desires, because they're stronger!

* You can, and indeed must, direct the "inner" you. The secret is to state repeatedly your positive affirmations, and to **strongly** visualise the slim you.

* Directing the "inner you" is the secret of success The stronger you make the image of the new you, the more certain is your success.

* Your beliefs about yourself and the world are picked up, often at random, from people you happen to meet, articles you happen to read, TV programmes you happen to see. They condition your mind to expect certain outcomes.

* Inner Slimming also conditions your mind—but this time **you** do the conditioning for an outcome that you want. You control you—maybe for the first time.

Once you start to direct your own mind, you have something far stronger than will power on your side. You have imagination and belief. With these, you can't fail.

But the body also affects the mind!!

Having, I hope, convinced you that successful slimming is not only in the mind, but controlled by the mind, let me show that the opposite is also simultaneously true.

Most people assume you can only change your attitude of mind through mental effort.

Let's take depression. Surely that's a purely mental state? Well, visualise someone who's depressed. What do you picture?

Shoulders slumped, eyes downcast, shallow breathing, low mumbled tone of voice, sagging muscles, mouth turned down. But these are all physical representations—and we just agreed that depression was purely mental!

The truth is that, whilst your mind does determine how your body behaves, equally how your body acts has an immediate impact upon your mental attitude.

It's a continuous loop.

YOUR OWN CONTINUOUS LOOP OF MIND AND BODY CONTROL

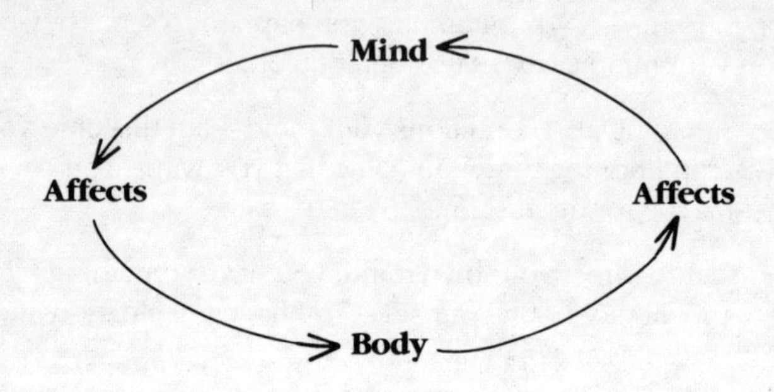

Let's experience an example.

Sit up straight. Put your shoulders back. Breathe deeply and tighten your chest and stomach muscles. Hold your head up, jaw muscles slightly tightened. Look ahead. Now smile. Make a purring noise of pleasure.

What do you feel? Alert? Capable? Confident? It works without fail. You changed your state of mind in seconds through actions.

It's the same with being slim. To be naturally slim you do need to think slim, but you also need to **act** slim. Then you'll get the natural commitment to be slim.

Watch a slim woman, someone you know perhaps, or a TV or movie personality. She walks confidently, she holds her body well, she holds her head well. All those signals are constant reinforcing messages to her mind to eat on a 1–5 basis. No will power involved, just confidence producing control.

The truth, as any professional actor will tell you, is that you can become confident by acting confident, you can become happy by acting happy. You can become slim by acting slim.

So think slim, act slim and you'll become slim.

Start putting in place your own continuous loop.

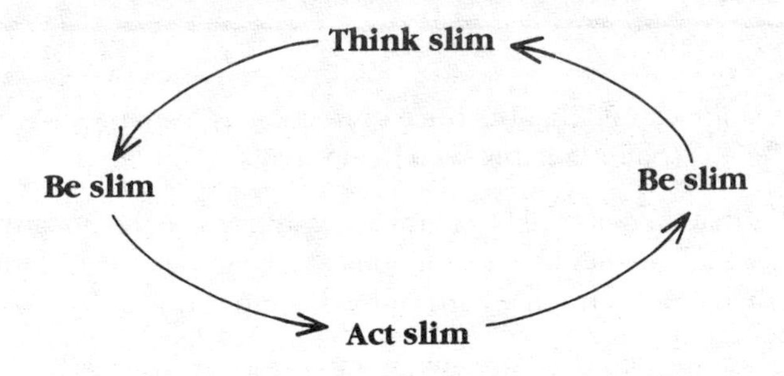

Now let's look at some typical situations where what happens in the mind and what happens to the body are completely linked together.

"It's knowing I can always be the weight I want. It's so ***easy,*** *that's the remarkable thing."*

Mandy Shires, Miss UK,
who slimmed 28 lbs in 6 weeks
—and won the title

THE EATING TRAPS

A Statesman once said that the price of freedom is eternal vigilance. There is some similarity with being slim!

The fact is that there are all too many traps into which the unwary slimmer can fall. Rather like the old idea of a bear trap, these traps are usually baited with some hard-to-resist temptations!

So let's examine some of these eating traps and then discuss how to cope with them.

Although I prefer the idea of an eating trap because it bring to mind a rather amusing (and accurate) picture, in fact psychologists call them eating "cues".

Either way, they are events or situations that trigger you wanting to eat—even though you're not actually hungry.

1. The Seefood" diet trap

This is the diet where, if you see food, you eat it! This trap is so obvious that it's easy to overlook it. The fact is that we really do often eat with our eyes. The more you see, the more you want.

If you keep food in sight, in the kitchen or in the living room, you'll definitely eat more.

Having food around, so that you're constantly reminded of it, is a sure way to start "grazing". Grazing is that "mind in neutral" state where you absent-mindedly munch your way through a whole bowl of peanuts without realising it.

Conclusion: Make an absolute resolution to keep food completely out of sight except at meal time.

2. The "I've been good all day and haven't eaten a thing" trap

This is a variation of the grim "all or nothing" approach.

Doris works hard. In fact, she rarely, if ever, has breakfast, and as often as not skips lunch.

Nor surprisingly, she comes home at about 6.30 feeling exhausted and hungry.

By 7 o'clock, despite her "will power", she's bored and desperate for something sweet to eat, because she knows she feels better when she's had some chocolate. So she eats the chocolate—but an hour later feels hungry again. She goes into the kitchen, sees the biscuit tin, and eats some biscuits while she prepares "something worthwhile".

Having eaten a meal, she has a dessert and rounds it all off with a mini binge just before bedtime.

Here's what went wrong:

Your physical hunger is, to a large extent, determined by your blood sugar level. After you eat a well-balanced meal, your blood sugar level will gradually rise. When it's high, you don't feel hungry.

Then, over the subsequent hours, it will gradually drop. When it's low, you feel hungry. If it drops too low, you start to feel ravenous and you're ready to binge.

By not eating all day, Doris had allowed her blood sugar level to drop really low and was setting herself up for a frenzied attack on the chocolate biscuits!

But that was only Mistake No.1. Mistake No.2 was the way she tackled her hunger. She went for the sweet foods.

Now the fact is that eating sugary foods—sweets, colas, biscuits, chocolate bars, etc.—will result in a more rapid rise in your blood sugar level. But because the rise is short and sharp, something undesirable happens. Your pancreas is automatically stimulated to produce insulin. The insulin gets into your bloodstream and has the effect of lowering your blood sugar level. As your blood sugar level drops, you start to feel hungry again.

That's why eating what are called the simple carbohydrates—the sugar-rich foods—can lead to so many problems. It's a "quick fix" —and as a normal way to cure hunger pains, it's storing up trouble.

Why? Well, first of all you're inviting a roller-coaster reaction. Feel hungry/eat sweets/quick rise in blood sugar level/quick insulin response to damp it down/feel hungry again. And so the cycle continues.

It can be worse. Over a period of months or years, your body may adapt to this cycle and you begin to maintain a higher than normal level of insulin. So when you do eventually go on a low-sugar diet, your body starts to react badly, you get in a foul mood, feel lethargic and soon break the diet.

And it can be much worse. After years of triggering an insulin response to constant snacking on high-sugar foods, your body may start to fail to produce enough insulin. The result of that is that you can suffer continuously high blood sugar levels—and that can lead to a type of diabetes, which is highly undesirable.

Well, I make no apologies for the short medical lesson, because we're learning some important facts here.

Fact 1

Sugar-rich foods give you a "quick fix" because they quickly raise your blood sugar level, but the results are only temporary and can be harmful in the long term.

Fact 2

Foods containing what are called complex carbohydrates—rices, pasta, grains, bread, etc—are converted to sugar more slowly in your body. So they satisfy you longer and don't over-stimulate your insulin production.

Fact 3

The best solution is to keep your blood sugar at a moderate level all the time. And the best way to do that is to eat little and often.That's why you always read that it's important to have breakfast and not to skip lunch. Eating little and often is exactly what our primeval ancestors did—and they never had a weight problem!

Your own "high-risk" situations

If we continue to think of situations tht trigger 6–10 eating as traps to catch the unwary, then it's obvious that some situations are more high-risk than others!

Everyone has their own individual traps. To identify yours, why not:

a. think back to the situations that triggered "semi-conscious" eating and note them down;

b. review your feedback chart and look for patterns that emerge. These will be your personal high-risk food traps

   Some typical ones might be:

   seeing a TV food commercial

   a regular meeting with someone who irritates you

   walking past the baker's or the hamburger bar

   watching TV and snacking

   a buffet

   a tempting dessert—even when you're full!

Have you made your own eating trap list? If so, we will take a break to review an important aspect of motivation, and then discuss tactics to avoid the traps.

There's no such thing as failure!

I really believe there is no such thing as failure. There are only results. Some results are what you want, some are **not** what you want. So you need a different approach.

Thomas Edison tried over 1000 prototypes before he finally invented the electric light bulb. When asked how he could keep going in the face of so much failure, he replied: "But I didn't fail: I just discovered 999 ways of **not** making a light bulb." So each time he was nearer the ultimate solution.

Now most of us don't think like that. We take on every mistake as emotional baggage, weighing us down.

Why not look at things another way? Being overweight, for example, is not a failure. It's simply that you followed a set of actions that produced a result—a result called excess fat. All you need to do is learn to follow a different set of actions to produce a new result—a result called being slim.

And that's what this six weeks will achieve for you.

> *"Thinking is the hardest work there is.*
> *That's why so few people do it!"*
> Henry Ford

BE A FREEDOM (FROM FAT) FIGHTER!

We've talked this week about situations that trigger unnecessary eating. We called them "eating traps". Now let's see how we can avoid them.

It's all part of what most people call the "battle of the bulge". Indeed, there are a lot of military terms involved in dieting—you "fight" temptation, and embark on a diet "campaign".

Well, if it is war, the way to win it is through guerilla tactics—not an all-out assault.

Instead, let's resolve to employ a number of subtler tactics. Become a Freedom Fighter—a Freedom From Fat Fighter. Tell your friends you're on the guerilla diet!

Avoiding Eating Traps

If you check your list of 'eating traps' one thing is certain to come through. You have some eating habits that are frequently, if not always, linked to 6–10 type eating, i.e. semi-conscious, unnecessary calorie consumption.

The association, the link, may be something simple—like watching TV and eating snack food. Or eating dinner and reading. The trick is to break the link—break the association. When you break the association, you break the trigger for semi-conscious, unnecessary eating and you regain control.

There's a further interesting reason why the link between, say, eating and watching TV or eating and reading is so powerful. Generally speaking, the activity you have linked to eating is pleasurable. So this feeling of enjoyment comes to be associated in your mind with eating and, in this way, watching TV or reading becomes subconsciously associated with eating—**not because you are necessarily hungry.**

TACTIC NO. 1
Eat in one place—and don't do anything else!

We've agreed that you must really concentrate on eating, so you taste the calories rather than waste the calories. And the best way is to set aside one place only to eat. This way, you associate eating with nothing else but the food you eat.

If it feels awkward at first, it's a sure sign that you are indeed associating your eating with another activity.

For lots of us—myself included—it may have been coming home from work and eating in front of the TV. When we stopped and ate together in the kitchen or dining room, we found we enjoyed the fact of unwinding by talking together— and were genuinely surprised at how much more we enjoyed the food.

If your partner or family demur—tell them why. After all, if it's a bad habit for you to eat and do something else—it's a bad habit for them too. And you certainly want to ensure that your children acquire the skill of being naturally slim early on.

Clearly the eating/TV link is only just one example. Others might be eating/reading, eating/phoning, eating/hobby. Whatever the link—**break** it. It really matters.

This most definitely includes eating/motoring. There's no way you can savour something and drive at the same time!

TACTIC NO. 2
Eat slowly

Yes, I know you've heard it lots of times before—but this time I'm going to remind you exactly why.

An important part of your brain is the hypothalamus. This controls a mechanism that some diet researchers call the appestat. Effectively, it's the function of the brain that regulates your hunger. It signals you to eat, and it signals you to stop eating when you are satisfied. It's a bit like the thermostat that switches your central heating on and off.

If your thermostat is triggered by a rise or fall in temperature, what triggers your appestat?

A similar rise and fall occurs, but this time in your blood sugar level. If your blood sugar level is low you "feel" hungry and your appestat is switched on—so you want to eat.

If your blood sugar level rises, your appestat is switched off and you want to stop eating. So it makes sense to let the appestat work sensitively.

What causes your blood sugar level to rise? When your body metabolises the food you eat into sugar. This then passes into the blood stream.

Now it makes sense that this takes a little time—about 20 minutes. Consequently, if you bolt your food down with scarcely a pause, the metabolic process can't possibly work fast enough to send a message to the appestat. So the first message your body gives you is that tight feeling in your skirt or belt!

That's hardly a fine-tuned signal! Result—you're in the 6–10 danger zone before you know it.

If, however, you eat slowly, with plenty of pauses, you'll find that your body will give you the right signals. You'll be aware. You are, in a phrase that you should really take into your permanent vocabulary, "listening to your body". Then you'll find it easy to stop eating at 5 on the Hunger-Meter scale—because your appestat tells you.

So Tactic No. 2 is to eat slowly.

Now I must admit that, previously, I could have qualified for the Olympic speed eating event! If you too have that problem, here's four ideas that work.

a. Put your fork down between bites. If it's in constant motion, you'll never slow down enough to stop at 5!

b. Stop and have a sip of water after every two or three bites. It breaks the rhythm and actually fills you up too!

c. Make a few real pauses in the meal—and check your imaginary Hunger-Meter. Are you at 3, 4, 5 or even 6? The more you pause to listen to your body, the more you become aware of how your stomach feels. The easier it is to stop when you're pleasantly satisfied.

d. Actually stop and touch your stomach. If you want to become aware, to focus on any one part of your body, the natural thing to do is to touch it. So lightly touch your stomach during your meal.

It's an absolute fact that the faster you eat, the more likely you are to put on weight. So slow down. The bonus is that you'll notice your food more and get more pleasure from it.

TACTIC NO. 3
Be calm

I well remember the circumstances of the most expensive meal out my wife and I ever had. Half way through we had an "upset". It didn't last long, but we both remarked on the same thing afterwards—we literally never tasted the second half of the meal. What a waste of money!

But there's an important truth here. If you eat when you're angry, or upset, or distracted—you don't really taste what you eat.

And if you don't taste the calories, you waste the calories.

Moreover, if you're distracted you'll go on eating long after your body has started giving you signals to stop.

The only way to ensure your eating is conscious eating is to be calm when you eat.

How? Well, there are two tactics you can employ. The first is to wait until the distraction is over. Attack the problem with your mind, not your fork!

The second—and I really recommend it—is to take some slow, deep, relaxing breaths in a particular way. I'll explain how shortly.

TACTIC NO. 4
Wise buys

Whilst we don't believe that any food should be on your forbidden list—because it only makes it obsessional—it's obvious that if you simply don't have calorie-rich, nutrition-poor foods in your larder, you can't eat them.

So tactic No. 4 is simple but effective. Avoid buying the really fat-laden, sugar-laden foods when you shop. Then you can't eat them later!

TACTIC NO. 5
Riding the wave

A diet expert I admire recently compared our food cravings to a wave. Most people think that the urge to eat, or eat something specific, builds up and builds up until, in the end, it has to be satisfied—like a wave will ultimately crash down on the beach. But there's a perfectly good alternative.

Instead of passively waiting to be engulfed by that wave—that craving to eat—you can actually outlast it. You can, as it were, surf on it. Because the truth is that you can nearly always outlast a craving and it will subside. Hunger will actually disappear if you wait. Try it and see!

However, you are unlikely to outlast it by just sitting around thinking about the food in question!

So the tactic is to start doing something that requires your concentration and attention. It takes a lot less control to start doing something else than to stop thinking of food!

We found the most helpful thing to do is to make a list **in advance.** Have it in the kitchen, and when an unwelcome craving occurs (one that you don't want to satisfy with a small portion), go to the list and start some activity that diverts your attention. The wave will subside surprisingly soon. You'll feel really good that you succeeded. You won. You were in control.

You must make your own list of alternative activities, but it might include:

Telephoning a friend	Shopping for a magazine
Working on a hobby	Doing some gardening
Reading a book	Visiting someone
Going out for a walk	Playing a game
Doing a crossword puzzle	etc. etc.

TACTIC NO. 6
One portion at a time

Another obvious help in acquiring more control over your eating is not to serve yourself more than one helping at a time.

If you make one piece of toast at a time, for example, you're a little less likely to go back and make a second piece.

If you serve half your normal portion first, there will be occasions when you finish the first half, pause, and realise you really don't need the second half. That you've reached '5' already.

I can assure you that the first time you do this you'll get a super sense of achievement. A confident feeling of being in **control.**

So make this tactic work for you. It's deceptively powerful.

TACTIC NO. 7
Keep food out of sight

Our eyes are most definitely bigger than our stomachs!

For most people, the sight of food is the most powerful stimulus of all to starting eating.

Make it a rule to **always** put food away. Put it in the cupboard or in containers. If it's out and can be picked at—it will be!

And be aware of those seductive TV food commercial and magazine ads. And shop windows. And cooking smells.

Keeping food out of sight—and keeping out of sight of food—is a simple BUT VITAL tactic until your new control becomes fixed enough.

I think the image of a Freedom Fighter is a good one. Freedom Fighters usually have a rather romantic image. They fight for a just cause and they employ subtle tactics!

That's just what we need to do. If you follow the ideas in this book, you genuinely will be free. You will never have to go on a diet again—in the sense of depriving yourself. Dieting will cease to be an issue in your life because you will have full control over your relationship with food. You'll control it—not vice versa. Freedom from FAT!

Isn't that worth fighting for?

So let's end this section with the Ten Commandments of the true Freedom Fighter. The Ten Commandments that will triumph in the battle of the bulge!

THE TEN COMMANDMENTS OF THE FREEDOM FIGHTER

1. Eat in one place

2. Do nothing else

3. Eat slowly

4. Be calm when you eat

5. Buy wisely

6. Ride the wave! (outlast the urge)

7. One portion at a time

8. Keep food out of sight!

Finally, add the two most important of all:

9. Eat only at 1–5 on the Hunger Meter

10. Eat only 6–10 foods

RELAX – AND SLIM

This has been a busy week, so an invitation to relax should be very welcome!

Relaxation is a major help to any slimmer. Remember, we have already agreed that stress is very fattening. And we certainly don't want to use food to calm ourselves!

Instead, I wholeheartedly recommend the following deep breathing method. If you've never tried deep breathing, you will be astonished at how quickly it can relax you and bring about a wonderful sense of peace and calm. In addition, the same type of deep breathing increases the flow of oxygen to the brain and makes you more alert. It is the breathing used in the practice of meditation, in yoga and in relaxation during childbirth. It's no accident we talk about the "breath of life".

DEEP BREATHING TO GROW CALM

Place your hand over your navel and imagine you have a balloon in your stomach. Breathe deeply through the nose, filling the balloon. Feel the balloon inflate and move your hand outwards. The further your hand moves, the deeper you have drawn air into the bottom of your lungs. Breathe as deeply as possible but without overbreathing. If you find breathing difficult through the nose, breathe through your mouth, but always draw the air into the bottom of the lungs.

As you breathe out, imagine the balloon deflating and feel the abdomen falling. Your out-breath should take longer than inhaling, and be accompanied by a slight sigh, because this sigh also helps to release tension.

After breathing in, hold the breath for 2 to 4 seconds, then exhale and again hold the breath for 2 to 4 seconds. Become aware of this precise moment of stillness and how easily the mind can focus on a single idea. Also remember this quiet relaxed moment when you are next in a stressful situation.

If you practise slow, deep breathing, you will also find that your ability to relax increases and your heart rate will decrease.

You can reach a wonderful relaxed state with the following simple procedure:

1. Imagine the balloon in your abdomen. Feet it inflate when breathing in, feel it deflate when breathing out.

2. Breathe in. Be aware of the air flowing in as the balloon inflates.

3. Breathe out gently, with a long sigh as the balloon deflates. Expel the air fully.

4. Pause.

5. Breathe in. Be aware of the air filling your lungs.

6. Hold it.

7. Breathe out with a sigh. Feel the warm air leave your body. Expel the air totally.

8. Pause.

9. Breathe in. Be aware of the air flowing in.

10. Hold it.

11. Breathe out with a sigh and feel the tension draining away.

12. Pause.

If you resolve to take ten of these deep breaths three times a day, you will experience a wonderful improvement in your energy level, your sense of well-being and your health.

* This simple breathing exercise is taken from the book *Accelerated Learning*

FEEDBACK CHART – WEEK FOUR

Day	Time	Hunger Scale 1–10 Start	Finish	What I ate	Food Scale 1–10	What I felt	Sat Down	I was calm/ composed	Savoured it

My assessment of Week Four is:
(Write your suggested corrective action)

My assessment of myself on the 1—10 commitment scale is:

I exercised 3 times a week for a 20 minute minimum period Yes

PARTICIPATION

What I learned this week

What I agreed with

Things I disagree with. Why?

N.B. Don't spectate—participate. Fill in your Feedback Chart each week, and when you've completed it, review it and write down any conclusions you come to. Remember, the skill of being slim has nothing to do with will power—but everything to do with motivation.

THE MIND & BODY DIET™

WEEK FIVE

DEALING WITH FEARS

Fear of success

I hope you're ready for this, but the truth is that, for some people, success in slimming can be a bit threatening!

You see, being overweight does have some benefits. It's a good—even if normally subconscious—excuse.

* There's the "I'll get a part-time job when I've lost the weight" syndrome. As the person approaches the realisation of that goal, he or she suddenly sees the excuse melting away with the fat.

* There's the "I'm just one of the girls" syndrome. Some women, who enjoy a comfortable 'non-competitive' relationship with other women, suddenly find their new-found attractiveness takes some adjusting to. They are seen differently by both men and women. And whilst it will eventually be a wonderful boost to their self-confidence, short term it can be a bit scary. Especially if they start getting some compliments from the opposite sex.

* It's true, too, that being overweight can help some people avoid relationships or situations they are nervous of—social situations, for example, or sports, or parties or dating. For them, it's necessary to face the real challenge, otherwise their conscious mind will say "lose weight", while their subconscious will say "stay fat".

  In our society, having sexual feelings and even admitting them to yourself is too often repressed. It is not at all uncommon for women and men to "opt out" of the challenges of sexual relationships by becoming overweight.

  As with all problems, the only way is to think it through, decide whether it could apply to you, and decide to handle the situation other than by eating. Unless you do, the mind will continue to look for ways to maintain the old defence—of being overweight.

* Many people need to take time getting used to their new, attractive figure. We are, unfortunately, all too often trained to make light of our successes. That's wrong. Take the credit. You, and only you, are responsible for your slimming success. The Uni-Vite products make slimming simple—but they don't make it easy. It's **your** effort and commitment that are bringing results.

  Similarly, this book only provides advice. It's your determination that puts it into practice. These are only the tools: the result is yours. Faced with a work of art, you don't praise the paints—you praise the artist!

  So feel good about your successes. If you look more attractive, be proud. If people compliment you, acknowledge that it took some effort, but it was worth it. Say: "I **do** feel good". Self-confidence and self esteem is your biggest guarantee of remaining slim for life.

* There are other people who are apprehensive about success—people who find they were noticed because of their size. When they lose the weight, this form of physical status is less important. This is more common with men. Indeed, we even use the expression "a big man" to denote someone in a powerful position.

* Another, quite common, experience can be a slight "let down" feeling as you near target weight.

  It may have been such a challenge that you are left wondering what to do now. After all, a challenge in life is often more exhilarating than the final goal! The answer is to set a new goal in your life. It's more than likely that the skills you've learned here will help. After all, slimming is not an end in itself.

* The other reality is that some people expect that reaching the ultimate goal of slimness will bring them all the things they've ever wanted. A new job, perhaps, or a new partner. Almost certainly it will help but, by itself, it may not be enough. So you need to be realistic and treat getting slim and remaining slim as one of life's important goals, not the only one.

* There's a final, subtle fear at work too. Once you find out that losing weight on the low-calorie/high-nutrition programme is really rather quick and simple, then you do have to admit to yourself that you were responsible for becoming overweight in the first place. You have no excuse now to fail—which is not so easy to admit!

  Along with the knowledge that it's possible to control your weight comes the responsibility to do so.

Fear of failure

There is a common experience of reaching a weight plateau just before finally achieving target weight. Sometimes—however illogical it may sound—it's caused by the fear of regaining weight once the target is ultimately attained!

You see, lots of people have been on a diet only to find they later regained the weight. They then felt a failure—even ashamed. So they don't want to experience that feeling again.

The answer to this fear is contained in both the low-calorie/high-nutrition diet range—and in this book.

The Uni-Vite diet will enable you to act quickly if you put on 3–4 lbs. Because that's the danger signal. If you don't put on 3 lbs, you can't put on 3 stone. The time to act is immediately. Put a mark on your scales 4 lbs over your target weight and ACT if you hit that mark.

This book is giving you the skills you need to cope mentally with the realities of life. The reality is that lapses will occur, and that you will get periods of stress and self doubt.

The reality, too, is that most people do put weight back on—because they haven't learned what you are learning. They haven't learnt the secret of LARA.

And LARA stands for?

L earning the skill of being slim
is to be **A** ware of what you do when something goes wrong
and **R** eview it without self criticism
then **A** ct to correct it

Look at it this way. If you put on weight as a result of stress, it's no different from developing a headache. Yet you wouldn't be ashamed of getting a headache.

So there's no shame in previous failures—the only failure is not to face up to a bit of self-analysis, admit you are responsible and take action!

MOTIVATION

The most motivated people I know are realistic. They want to know the facts, so they can make up their own minds. You need to be convinced before you become committed.

Researchers into weight loss have discovered three factors that characterise successful slimmers:

Three predictors of success

1. Your chances of long-term weight maintenance are doubled if you reach your target weight. Not "almost"—but exactly. That's why it's important to follow the Uni-Vite Personalised Diet Plan while you're also following this 6 week course, and to continue to follow it all the way down to the goal weight that you and your doctor have set.

2. Your chances of long-term weight maintenance are tripled if you consciously raise your exercise level. The type of exercise is virtually immaterial—**walking is just fine!**

   It's not just the calories you burn or the increase in your metabolism you achieve—although both are vital. It's the simple fact that the people who exercise are more committed.

   Think about it!

3. Your chances of long-term weight maintenance are related to the number of "get out clauses" you allow yourself.

   What's a "get out" clause? **It's basically the number of times you're prepared to excuse yourself in advance!**

   I'm not extolling the virtues of an "all or nothing" approach to dieting. That—as we have seen—is setting yourself up to fail. Because all or nothing always ends in nothing!!

   What I am saying is that the fewer built-in excuses you make, the more likely you are to succeed.

Here's a list of some typical "get out" clauses. How far down the list would you say was reasonable?

Typical get-out clauses

I'm prepared to ignore my diet programme:-

1. On Christmas Day
2. On a family celebration/birthday
3. When we're entertaining
4. When we're on holiday
5. At a party
6. When we're out for a meal
7. When visitors call
8. When cakes are passed around at an office celebration
9. So I don't offend friends
10. When I've cooked a Sunday lunch
11. When we're out at the pub
12. At a business lunch
13. Not to waste the food I've paid for
14. When I'm busy

What other get-out clauses can you think of? How far down the list should you go before you begin to betray a lack of commitment? A lack of motivation?

KNOWLEDGE IS ESSENTIAL IF YOU ARE TO BE CONVINCED ....
CONVICTION IS ESSENTIAL IF YOU ARE TO BE COMMITTED

The remainder of this week is devoted to facts—facts that will help to convince you that your determination to slim is right, and that nothing less than full commitment will do.

You'll learn that:

* Once a fat cell is created, it can shrink, but it won't disappear.
* An "apple" shape is a danger sign.
* Most overweight people skip breakfast.
* There is a "body set point".
* Fat children tend to become fat adults.
* Your basal (basic) metabolism accounts for most of the calories you burn. But exercise can boost it.
* Many overweight people really **do** have a slower metabolism than the naturally slim—but that's a fact, not an excuse.
* All diets slow down your metabolism temporarily—only exercise keeps it up whilst you slim.

  The amount of calories you burn is related to your body size. So if you lose weight you are smaller, and if you are smaller you **must** consume less calories.

FAT FACTS

Fat cells

Diet researchers believe that when you put on weight—especially as a child—the number of fat cells increases. But in addition, the size of your fat cells also expands. More fat cells and bigger fat cells!

When you lose weight, only the size of your fat cells shrinks—the number remains constant.

In other words, they are always lurking there ready to pounce! That's why it's vital to learn the skill of being slim.

Apples or pears?

It's not just how much extra weight you carry, it's where the fat is deposited that counts—especially in relation to your health.

Men tend to put fat on in their belly area. They become apple shaped. Women tend to deposit fat on their thighs, buttocks and hips—the pear shape.

Now women may resent it, but in fact it's more difficult to lose fat from thighs, buttocks and hips than from your stomach. On the other hand, "apples" have a far greater risk of heart disease than "pears".

The rule is simple. For men, a waist that's bigger than their hips is a danger sign. A signal that you are at risk.

If a woman has a waist that is only just smaller than her hips, then that is also a danger sign. She, too, is at risk.

So if you have a pot belly or beer belly, act now. It's not the jolly sign it may have seemed.

Most overweight people don't eat breakfast!

It's all too easy to get smug—you don't have breakfast and then get ravenous later. A little and often is what our bodies want.

Hunger is not a virtue—it only encourages pent up bingeing.

The body set point theory

Many researchers believe that, after you have been at a certain weight for some time, the body tends to resist change.

So if you lower your body weight, there's a stubborn tendency for the body to want to return to the original weight.

That's why it's essential, when you've reached your target weight, NOT to gleefully relax and assume the battle is won.

A few weeks of continuing to review all the advice, a commitment to exercise, and a determined effort to incorporate the low-calorie/high-nutrition foods into your lifestyle, will ensure that your body adjusts to a new set point.

The one you want!

Fat children become fat adults

Parents have an awesome responsibility in determining whether their children will struggle with the pounds, or sail through life envied as "naturally slim".

Consider these statistics:

a. 75% of children who are fat between the ages of 9–12 grow up to be fat adults.

b. 90% of fat adolescents grow to be fat adults.

c. Breast-fed babies are slimmer. If the mother can see there's some milk left in the bottle, she tends to feed the baby till it's all gone—even though the baby may not have wanted it all. That sets up habits of over-eating.

d. Parents who habitually eat fat-laden excess meals, or eat too fast, pass those traits on.

e. Parents who commonly use food as a reward, or to comfort hurt feelings, teach an association between food and mood—not food and need.

f. Parents who do not encourage exercise encourage inactivity. Inactivity is a very strong predictor of excess weight.

ALL ABOUT METABOLISM

1. The three ways you burn calories

It used to be thought that the average woman needed 2100 calories a day to maintain a constant weight. Now, as we have seen —owing to more sedentary lifestyles—it's nearer 1850.

That 1850 calories burned comes from three sources.

a. The first is your basal metabolism—the energy you need to keep your body ticking away. That's about 1 calorie a minute —1400 a day. It's constant, even if you're lying around doing nothing. You'll see it represents about 75% of your energy expenditure.

b. The second way you use energy is via work and/or exercise. This varies according to the intensity of the exercise. So, for example, light housework burns $2\frac{1}{2}$ calories a minute, brisk walking burns 4 calories a minute, and heavy manual labour burns 7 calories a minute.

   For most of us, exercise represents about 20% of our energy expenditure.

c. The third way we burn calories is by eating! It's called the thermogenic response to food. (Thermo = heat, genic = creating). Most of us experience a rise in temperature when we eat or drink too much. That's our body trying to burn off the excess calories. Not always successfully if we overload it!

d. Now many women will be interested to know that, in a pregnant woman, this thermogenic response is suppressed, because her body is deliberately trying to conserve energy.

   However, the same thing happens when she's on the pill, because the pill works by "fooling" her body into thinking she's already pregnant.

So the thermogenic response doesn't work well for a woman who's on the pill—the act of eating doesn't trigger a rise in temperature or an increase in metabolism. Consequently, women on the pill will burn slightly fewer calories.

2. Laughter increases your metabolic rate!

So laugh and grow slim!

3. A woman's metabolism drops just after her period

She should feel less hungry then. A good time to reduce calorie intake.

In contrast, she will feel more hungry and more like eating carbohydrate during the second half of her period—as the level of the hormone progesterone rises.

4. You can rely on your metabolism

The human body is an exquisitely balanced mechanism. Left to itself, its natural tendency is to maintain itself in balance.

The truth for most people is that, if you genuinely "listened to your body" and didn't override its signals, you would never put weight on! The trouble, as we've seen, is that we eat because it's lunchtime or because the food looks good, or because we're angry. And we often start at 4 or even 5 on the Hunger-Meter. If only we checked before we started to eat and asked a simple question — "Do I really need this?"—hardly any of us would ever have a weight problem.

The more we pay genuine attention to our feelings of fullness, the easier it is to be naturally slim. Your real feelings are a far better guide to when to start and stop eating than all the boring calorie charts ever devised.

Here's a fact to ponder on. Naturally slim people don't have any more will power than overweight people—but they have more confidence. Confidence in their own feelings of when to start and stop eating.

5. Many overweight people really do have a slower metabolism than the naturally slim

So you needn't feel guilty BUT—we've said before—having a low metabolism is a reason, not an excuse!

It may be unfair that you can't eat as much as your skinny friend without putting weight on—but if it's a fact, you have to adjust to it.

And that's what this six weeks is all about.

6. Your metabolism does drop when you go on any calorie-restricted diet

It's nature's way of conserving energy—even if it's not helpful! The reduction, however, is no more and no less just because you are on a low-calorie diet.

The only way to keep your metabolic rate up whilst you are dieting is to exercise.

When you stop dieting on the Uni-Vite programme, your metabolism will go back up to normal after a week or two. If you want to increase your metabolism long-term, i.e. burn more daily calories, then you need to increase the amount of "lean mass"—i.e. muscle—in your body. The only way to do that is through exercise.

7. Your metabolism is related to your size

It's obvious, if you think about it, that carrying weight around uses energy. So the bigger you are, the more calories you burn, and vice versa. That's why men need more calories than women—and why they lose weight easier.

But it also explains why you must reduce your calorie intake after you've lost weight—otherwise you are certain to put weight back on. In fact, you need 8 calories less for every lb you lose. So if you lose 30 lbs, you need to consume 240 calories less per day than you did at your previous weight.

That makes the last section this week rather important.

FAT ALERT!

I like the idea of "calorie trading"—in other words, "saving" calories on one day in order to "spend" them on an absolutely delicious meal another day.

The wise calorie trader, therefore, doesn't squander calories on 1–4 foods—foods with high calorie content and low nutritional value.

I find it MUCH simpler not to bother agonizing over the estimated calorie content of food. Instead, I have a simple list of high-fat foods. Since fat has over **twice** the calories, weight for weight, of protein or carbohydrate, the truth is that if you cut down on fat, this alone can be enough to stay slim. Fat is the real enemy.

The following chart gives you a list of the fat-rich foods to avoid, or at least cut back sharply. At the same time, reducing your fat intake reduces your risk of heart disease and strokes. Heart disease is the No. 1 killer in the UK, so you would be crazy not to.

The fat content in the average person's food accounts for about 900 calories a day of their energy intake!

It's **far** easier, and far more productive, to be conscious of your fat intake than to be obsessive about your calorie intake. So institute a "fat alert" campaign and ruthlessly cut down from today.

It's a lot easier to go easy on the list—(very easy at the top!)—than trying to count calories.

The clinching reason to reduce your intake of dietary fat is new evidence from Harvard University, noted by M S Leibman, Director of Nutrition at the American Centre for Science. It shows that a calorie of fat may be more fattening than a calorie of protein or carbohydrate. "The body appears to find it more efficient to produce body fat from dietary fat—it appears that the body converts fat in food directly to body fat".

FAT ALERT SCALE

This food	Has this much fat per ounce	And this many fat calories per ounce
A **whole day's** Uni-Vite food	3%	9 cals
Lard/vegetable oil	99%	254
Butter	82%	211
Margarine	81%	208
Mayonnaise	79%	205
French dressing	73%	187
Almonds	54%	167
Peanut butter	54%	178
Double cream	48%	127
Roast peanuts	49%	162
Cream cheese	47%	104
"Low" fat spread	41%	104
Grilled bacon	36%	104
Potato crisps	36%	110
Fresh coconut	36%	102
Sausage roll	36%	130
Cheddar cheese	34%	116
Pork sausage	32%	105
Fried onions	32%	105
Milk chocolate	30%	151
Pork pie	27%	107
Roast lamb	26%	100
Chocolate eclairs	25%	100

In praise of carbohydrate

There's a fallacy that carbohydrate is fattening. In quantity, it is—everything is except water! But you're far better off with wholemeal bread or pasta than a pork pie—assuming, of course, that you don't put anything more than a smear of low fat spread on the bread, and don't smother the pasta with cream.

THE HIDDEN PERIL

800–1000 calories a day. That's the number of calories the average person gets from fat in their regular diet. It's 38%–40% of the average person's calorie intake. Which means it's 50% or more of some people's daily diet! That's a crisis point!

Since this level of fat means consuming over 1/4 lb of pure fat every day, it takes some believing. The reason is that so much fat is hidden—lurking in foods you don't suspect! Sauces, cheese (over 50% fat), bacon, sausages, hamburgers, crisps, nuts, roasts, pies, cakes and pastries.

Don't be fooled by sausage or paté makers who claim 95% meat—they're allowed to include fat as meat!

And when you read labels that give you nutritional information per 100 grams, remember that fat has 9 calories per gram, **twice** as many as protein and carbohydrate, which have 4.

So if a label reads:		**It really means:**
Per 100 grams		*% of calories*
Protein	18g	12%
Carbohydrate	40g	26%
Fat	42g	62%
	—	—
Calories	610	100%

So how to cut down on this hidden peril?

* Steam or microwave vegetables and season with herbs and spices rather than sauces and butter.
* Cut out salad dressing—use yoghurt or lemon juice.

* Trim off all visible fat.
* Bread rolls genuinely taste better without butter—after you get used to the idea.
* Always use skimmed milk.
* Increase fish in your diet.
* Don't fry—ever. Grilled food tastes better.
* Use either oven-baked chips or brush your own chips lightly with oil and bake them. That saves half the calories! Ideally, switch to baked potatoes in their skins.
* Go easy on cakes, biscuits and croissants.
* Read labels!!

Fat footnote!

Here are some fascinating fat facts. "Fink" about them!

a. 4 oz of roast duck with skin — 384 calories
4 oz of roast duck without skin — 229 calories (40% less)

b. 4 oz of dark chicken with skin — 288 calories
4 oz of white chicken without skin — 197 calories (32% less)

c. 51% of the calories in Cheddar cheese come from fat
9% of the calories in cottage cheese come from fat

d. 40% of the calories in a piece of chocolate cake come from fat
3% of the calories in a piece of bread come from fat

e. 54% of the calories in streaky bacon come from fat
17% of the calories in a grilled pork chop come from fat

f. 54% of the calories in crisps come from fat
0% of the calories in an apple come from fat

FABULOUS FIBRE!

You'd have to have just returned from exile on a desert island not to know that fibre is "in".

But did you know that there's more than one type of fibre? And it does much more than improve regularity!

Most people still have a vague notion that fibre acts like some sort of internal cleanser. A bit like a benevolent Brillo pad.

Fibre is the part of a plant that is not broken down in digestion. It's the structure that gives the plant its shape. The insoluble fibre moves through our bodies largely unaltered. As it does, it absorbs water and this assists a comfortable movement of waste matter through the bowel.

Increase fibre intake and you **decrease** cancer of the colon and constipation.

Increase the type of soluble fibre, known as gums and pectin, found in fruit and oats and, most experts believe, you can measurably reduce cholesterol levels, and therefore the chance of heart disease and strokes.

Increase your intake of both types of fibre and you feel fuller and will eat less of the calorie-rich foods. Moreover, fibre doesn't contain calories.

Sold?

Increase these foods for more fibre

High soluble fibre/pectin foods are:

Muesli, oatmeal, chick peas, beans, wholemeal bread, apples, bananas, oranges, figs, prunes, lentils, pears, grapefruit.

High fibre vegetables are:

Potatoes in skins, celery, carrots, cauliflower, cabbage, broccoli, aubergine, green beans, peas, parsnips, spinach, tomatoes.

WHY IT'S WORTH MAKING GOOD FOOD CHOICES

There's a limit to the number of calories we can use without storing them as fat. Consequently, if you eat a lot of low-nutrition foods—foods with too much fat or sugar in them—you'll have used up the calories you have to "spend" on poor food choices. So you either overeat to make up the nutrient gap—or suffer a deficiency.

At the same time, food is both a pleasure and a very important part of socialising, so you will naturally want as many calories as pssible to "spend" on social occasions.

I have successfully controlled my weight for five years without once having to diet, and without once having to refuse any food I really wanted, through a simple strategy. Whenever I need to eat, but the meal has little social significance, I use a low-calorie/high-nutrition food. In my case, obviously, it is a Uni-Vite food. It frees up calories to "spend" on more important occasions.

If you want to forget dieting as an issue in your life, my advice is to consciously incorporate low-calorie/high-nutrition foods into your lifestyle. Think of them as 6–10 foods.

The foods that provide good nutrition in moderate calories are not difficult to remember. They are:

Fruits and vegetables
Wholegrain breads and cereals
Beans and pulses
Skimmed milk
Cottage cheese, medium fat cheese
Eggs
Chicken and turkey
Fish and seafood

If you start to think of your favourite-tasting foods that are also on the above list as 9's and 10's on your personal food scale, you'll begin instinctively to make good choices.

If you're trying to keep fat off, it's not logical to eat it! And when you know that sugar is the carbohydrate food most readily converted to body fat, it's not logical to eat much of that, either.

Action

1. Start visualising fat-laden foods and sugar-rich foods as 1's on your Food-o-Meter.
2. Create a new motto for yourself:

   I don't count calories—I make every calorie count!

"I'm walking on air! My confidence and self-esteem have soared higher than at any time in my life."

Patti Carlson, Bloomingdale, Illinois, who slimmed 7st 7lbs in 6 months

DON'T EAT TOO LATE

"Breakfast is the most important meal of the day."

"Don't eat immediately before going to bed."

Common enough advice—and certainly sound advice for the slimmer, but do you know why?

Meals taken early in the day have the effect of inducing peaks of hormonal activity in a way that fights fat. Conversely, if you eat late, the lower hormone levels essentially reduce the body's natural ability to metabolise fat.

The practical result is astonishing. Scientists at the University of Minnesota actually prepared a paper entitled "We are not only what we eat—but when we eat".

They reached this conclusion after an imaginative series of experiments in which one group of people were given a precisely measured 2000 calorie a day menu. They were instructed to eat only breakfast. The other group ate only dinner—but the same 2000 calories.

The "early eating" group lost an average of 1½ lbs a week, while the late eaters gained. These results were confirmed in a study conducted for the US Government at Natick, Massachusetts, where the direct effect of eating early in the day, rather than later, was 1 lb a week weight loss.

While we are obviously not proposing to cut out the evening meal—the main social meal in a modern life—it is clearly only common sense to ensure that we enjoy adequate breakfast and lunch and are careful when evening arrives.

WOULD YOU LIKE TO SAVE 100,000 CALORIES A YEAR?

What an offer! Cutting out 100,000 calories a year would prevent you putting on 28 lbs!

In fact you can do that by making some changes which, in themselves, are quite small but which—added up over one year—can be a huge saving and make it easy to keep off the weight. Since there are 3500 calories in 1 lb of extra body fat, you can potentially prevent 7 lbs of weight creeping on for every 24,000 calories you save.

Let's start with the one that requires the most effort.

Action	*Saving each time*	*Annual saving*
1. Cut out 1 teaspoon of sugar per cup (4 cups of tea/coffee a day)	20 cals per teaspoon 80 cals a day 560 cals a week	29,000 calories
2. Cut out 2 peanut snacks a week	324 cals a packet 648 cals a week	33,000 calories
3. You cut down from 2 pieces of toast with 1/2 oz butter per slice to $1\frac{1}{2}$ slices using low fat spread	140 cals per time (say 280 cals a week) if you have 2 breakfasts like this a week	14,000 calories
4. You use 3/4 tablespoon of cooking oil instead 2 tablespoons when you brown meat	158 cals each time (say twice a week) 320 cals a week	16,000 calories
5. Substitute skimmed milk for gold top on your cereal. Cut 5 oz milk serving to 3 oz.	65 cals a serving (say 3 times a week) 200 cals a week	10,000 calories

The above 5 simple actions could cut out 100,000 calories a year!

The point is that the saving each time is relatively small but, added up over a year, it's the difference between fat and slim.

You eat over 1000 meals a year—every time you take a little bit smaller portion, or little bit less fat, it all adds up.

More easy changes

Here's a short list of small, easy changes that bring big results over the months. All it needs is a bit of thought.

	Saving per time	***Possible savings per year***
1. Make mayonnaise with 2/3 yoghurt	67 cals	5,000 cals
2. Use yoghurt instead of cream to make raspberry fool	180 cals	3,000 cals
3. Use lemon juice instead of vinaigrette on salads	145 cals	7,000 cals
4. Grill food instead of frying	100 cals	15,000 cals
5. Use low cal tonic in 4 gins and tonics a week	40 cals a drink	8,000 cals
6. Drink $3\frac{1}{2}$ pints instead of 5 pints of beer a week	270 cals a week	14,000 cals
7. Use quark or fromage frais instead of soured cream	120 cals	7,000 cals
8. Use stock instead of butter or oil to sauté vegetables	60 cals	8,000 cals

Action

Think through your ideas of small changes with big, long-term payoffs.

Final Thought

This week has concentrated mainly on the physical facts that you need to know to make logical decisions about your lifestyle. The only conclusion you can come to is that to concentrate on severely reducing your fat intake is a much easier, and much less restrictive, course of action than bothering to count calories.

Do this, and consciously increase your use of low-calorie/high-nutrition foods, and you can genuinely forget dieting as an issue.

"I am literally half the man I used to be and look half the age!"

Ray Berry, Manchester,
who slimmed 10 stone in 9 months

FEEDBACK CHART – WEEK FIVE

Day	Time	Hunger Scale 1–10 Start	Finish	What I ate	Food Scale 1–10	What I felt	Sat Down	I was calm/ composed	Savoured it

My assessment of Week Five is:
(Write your suggested corrective action)

My assessment of myself on the
1—10 commitment scale is:

I exercised 3 times a week for a
20 minute minimum period Yes

PARTICIPATION

What I learned this week

What I agreed with

Things I disagree with. Why?

N.B. Don't spectate—participate. Fill in your Feedback Chart each week and when you've completed it review it and write down any conclusions you come to. Remember the skill of being slim has nothing to do with will power—but everything to do with motivation.

THE MIND & BODY DIET™

WEEK SIX

THIS IS THE END OF THE BEGINNING — NOT THE BEGINNING OF THE END

This is the start of Week Six. But it's not the beginning of the end of our course together—today is the first day of your new life!

The whole point of the Mind & Body Diet Programme is to get you to think about the issues involved in learning to be slim. We've agreed that being slim is a skill, and rather like learning to swim well or play tennis well, you need to learn the techniques that eventually make it easy.

Just as it would be impossible to learn to play tennis by just reading a book, so it's impossible to acquire the skill of being slim purely by reading this book.

You can only be instinctively slim by thinking about the issues we've raised, practising the techniques, and incorporating the advice into your lifestyle. If you do, you will be able to maintain an ideal weight for life, without exercising grim will power or self-denial.

The truth is you are not just trying to change your weight—you are trying to change your lifestyle. One without the other doesn't last long. The prize is that you won't just be slim—you'll have a fabulous sense of well-being, energy, optimism and control over your life!

A prize like that is worth the effort.

To assist you in acquiring your new lifestyle, let's start by acquiring some new perspectives!

A NEW PERSPECTIVE

I'm sure you've heard the story about the two shoe salesmen who were both sent to an underdeveloped country.

The first wired back to head office: "Fabulous opportunity—almost no one here wears shoes". The second also wired home, but his opinion was: "No chance of any business—almost no one here wears shoes."

It's the same difference in perception that prompts the comment that a church can be half full—or half empty. It all depends on how you see a situation. Yet how you look at things may not only be wrong, it can lead to making poor and even destructive decisions about your life.

In the field of education, for example, a simple incident early in life can cause a devastating limitation on a child's future. So an apparently unimportant early maths test, in which she happened to get a poor mark, might prompt a chance remark: "Of course, she's not very good at maths". Subconsciously, the child "internalises" that thought, starts believing that she isn't "good at maths", and proceeds to act consistently—i.e. she becomes poor at maths. Yet she really has the latent ability all the time. A twisted thought held her back from her full potential.

I have argued, in the book *Accelerated Learning,* that the limits to learning are largely self-imposed and that if we would (not could, but would) lift these limits, the change in us and our children would be dramatic. The tragedy is that the techniques to release that potential are not difficult. Indeed, they are laid out in the *Accelerated Learning* book.

The relevance to slimming is this. Too often, chance remarks or incidents get twisted in our minds to create negative ways of looking at things. Many people's main form of exercise is jumping to false conclusions! False conclusions create false beliefs, and these false beliefs hold us back.

Let's play a game, but a game with a serious purpose. I have listed below some common beliefs about food, dieting, being fat and your self-image. Then I have given you the truth behind those beliefs, and finally a way of re-stating the old beliefs in ways that will help you change your own attitudes, so that they become consistent with an "I–never–need–diet–again" mentality.

The game is this. The old belief is stated first. Then the truth. Then a new interpretation, which I suggest you should consider incorporating into your own lifestyle, if it's relevant to you. Cover up the second and third sections each time and see if you can work out the truth, and then the new interpretation, for yourself. Very often, you'll need to turn old beliefs on their head!

❖ ❖ ❖ ❖ ❖

OLD BELIEF: Overeating is bad.

FACT: People often overeat to cope with stress, anger and anxiety—i.e. they cover up their problems with food. That's not bad —that's simply a misguided response that many people learn. Moral judgements about eating are irrelevant.

NEW BELIEF: Overeating simply proves that I need to think of new, direct ways to cope with life.

❖ ❖ ❖ ❖ ❖

OLD BELIEF: I can't like myself when I'm fat, but I will like myself when I lose weight.

FACT: Your value as a person is based on much more than your weight. Comparison with other people is pointless. Being fat or thin is neither good nor bad—it's just a physical state.

NEW BELIEF: I like myself for all sorts of reasons—my eyes, legs, skin, hands, teeth, perhaps—or my intelligence, sense of humour, smile, honesty, kindness, creativity, dependability. You are much more than a body: you are a personality—a parent, a son, a daughter, friend, lover. All these things matter more than being fat.

Once you accept this, you've created a sound basis to like yourself even more when you **do** regain the slimness that is a natural right.

❖ ❖ ❖ ❖ ❖

OLD BELIEF: Overeating means I'm out of control.

FACT: Continuing to eat when you are already full is a sign of too much control! You are overriding your body's natural signals to stop eating.

NEW BELIEF: If I listen to my body and eat 1–5, I'll regain the instinctive weight control that nature gave me.

OLD BELIEF: Eating when I'm worried makes me feel better.

FACT: Any relief is (very!) temporary. It's usually followed by a heavy dose of self-criticism. Tackle your worries with your mind, not your teeth.

NEW BELIEF: I can cope with anxiety in a number of ways. I can take specific action on the problem. I can admit I'm scared. I may have to accept the situation, because life isn't always fair or because I really can't influence the outcome. Or, much more productively, I can tell myself: "This, too, shall pass".

A recent study showed that, of the things that people worry about:

80% never actually happened

10% were out of the person's control anyway

5% did happen, but the consequences were less devastating than feared.

Conclusion: 95% of all worries are pointless!

The basic truth about human life is that bad situations **do** change. The main thing to fear is fear.

There are many events over which you have little or no control but one key fact over which you have **total** control is the way you react. You always have a choice over this.

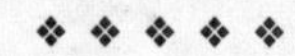

OLD BELIEF: Everyone notices me and thinks the less of me because I'm fat.

FACT: The blunt truth is that most people aren't all that interested in your appearance, any more than you are interested in theirs! They probably don't think of you as anywhere near as fat as you think you are, anyway. It's how you behave they remember.

NEW BELIEF: I am learning to be slim for my own sake, not because of some cultural "norm", or other people's reaction. My value as a person has nothing to do with my weight.

❖ ❖ ❖ ❖ ❖

OLD BELIEF: I recognise now that I eat when I'm angry—but if I express my anger openly, I'll be rejected.

FACT: People very commonly eat to try to dull their anger. The result is only to repress that anger—and sooner or later it will surface, often whilst you are losing the weight. You feel tense and angry without knowing why.

Expressing anger openly, but calmly and honestly, ALWAYS leads to a better relationship.

You cannot buy love by hiding your feelings.

NEW BELIEF: If I tell people firmly, but quietly, that they have hurt my feelings, or that they take me for granted, or that they have infringed my rights, they will listen much more than if I yell —and respect me for being honest.

* I can be angry—and still be loved
* I can be angry—and still be in control
* I can be angry—without being hurtful
* I can be angry—without being aggressive
* I have a right to express my feelings. And if I do, I'll eat less.

Don't say "yes" when you mean "no"! Express your anger in words—not food! It's a fundamental truth that when you express anger or hurt, it disappears. And as the anger in your mind disappears, so does the hunger in your stomach.

❖ ❖ ❖ ❖ ❖

OLD BELIEF: It's only right to clean my plate: waste not, want not. Wasting food is a sin.

FACT: Food has no moral value. Eating more than you need helps no one—not even the "starving millions".

NEW BELIEF: Leaving food is a sign that you recognise it has no magic properties. Food is purely your nourishment and enjoyment. When you reach 5—**stop!** In our society, food is, if anything, too readily available. So don't eat to prevent hunger—eat when you are hungry.

❖ ❖ ❖ ❖ ❖

OLD BELIEF: Eating when I'm lonely or bored makes me feel better

FACT: It doesn't for long! You only criticise yourself afterwards and feel bad about yourself. Life without pleasure is dull, but you can't expect to fill emotional gaps with food.

Everyone feels lonely or bored at some time. If you stop before you reach for the food and ask: "Why do I want to eat this?", you'll work out the real reason and be able to decide on an alternative course of action.

NEW BELIEF: I can differentiate between "mood" food and "need" food—between emotional hunger and physical hunger. I have alternatives, like calling a friend on the phone, involving myself in a hobby, going to the cinema, walking, deep breathing, relaxing with music, etc.

I can, indeed, get pleasure from the 6–10 foods I really love, but at the same time I will add other experiences to my life to enrich it and give me pleasure.

❖ ❖ ❖ ❖ ❖

OLD BELIEF: If I become slim, I'll be more sexually attractive. That could be a problem. I'm not sure I could handle the jealousy it might provoke, or the temptations it could bring. Being overweight helps me keep these issues at bay.

FACT: As long as your partner is confident of your feelings, he or she will be pleased with your appearance.

Your sexuality is an important part of your personality and can be expressed without inhibition.

NEW BELIEF: I can trust myself, and I have the right to say honestly what I want, or don't want, in my sexual life.

❖ ❖ ❖ ❖ ❖

OLD BELIEF: The fact that I've dieted before and put the weight back on proves I'm a failure.

FACT: You didn't fail—the diet did! The diet was at fault, not you.

NEW BELIEF: Conventional diets don't work for lots of reasons that I now know. I can succeed now because I understand how to reach the inner "me".

❖ ❖ ❖ ❖ ❖

OLD BELIEF: I need someone to "prod" me. Criticism is healthy.

FACT: We rebel against outside pressure to change. You have to want to change for yourself, not other people. Don't join any group where you'll be criticised for not losing weight. Criticism doesn't work. Caring, support and understanding does.

NEW BELIEF: I will change when I'm ready and for myself. Criticism, especially self-criticism, never produces anything except a poor self-image—and therefore more eating!

Self care works—self-criticism doesn't!

❖ ❖ ❖ ❖ ❖

OLD BELIEF: Some foods are good, some are bad.

FACT: If a food is a 10 for you, it's good—whatever the food. Psychologically, all foods are equal. If you deny yourself by eating what you "should", you'll only end up eating what you want in addition to what you should. Few people get a craving for a celery stick!

NEW BELIEF: No food is off limits for me—so long as I rate it 6–10 and really savour it. Of course, some foods are nutritionally much better for me, and this will influence my choice. I can have any food I want, but the question is: "Do I really want it?"

The more relaxed you are about food, the less you will eat.

❖ ❖ ❖ ❖ ❖

OLD BELIEF: It's lunch time—time to eat.

FACT: If you listen to your body, the only time to eat is when you're hungry. That could be 7 am, 9 am, 11 am, 12 noon, 3 pm or 5 pm.

NEW BELIEF: I can consciously tune in to my body and eat when it tells me, and as often as it tells me. Sometimes, that will be once a day: sometimes six times a day. That's the natural way to eat myself slim.

❖ ❖ ❖ ❖ ❖

OLD BELIEF: Chocolate is bad for me.

FACT: Different kinds of food provide different satisfactions.

For example, if you feel lonely, smooth or hot foods are more satisfying because they suggest warmth and comfort. They are soothing and remind us of childhood. Foods like ice cream, mousse, peanut butter, soup, milk, cocoa.

If you are angry, you are more likely to enjoy crunchy, hard, chewy foods that you use your teeth on (carrots, cereals, meat).

If you feel the need for love, or reward, chocolate provides a sensual satisfaction.

So the truth is that a little planned, savoured chocolate is not bad for you at all. If you **decide** that's what you really want, you'll eat less. However, you should be aware that chocolate contains a chemical that can be addictive.

NEW BELIEF: If I match my food to my mood, I will get more satisfaction and eat less.

So I'll think before I eat in future and make sure I get the maximum conscious pleasure from my food. I won't eat cheese when I really want apple pie, or fruit when I want chocolate. Not only will I savour what I eventually eat, but I will visualise the food I really want. I'll consider what texture it should be (liquid? creamy? chewy? smooth? crunchy?), what taste it should have (spicy? salty? sweet?) and whether it should be hot or cold.

This way, I'll get the maximum enjoyment out of what I eat, and I'll also eat less.

I hope you found the game of restructuring old beliefs interesting and thought-provoking.

Did you notice how often conventional wisdom was the opposite of the truth? How sweeping general conclusions are often drawn from single, untypical instances?

Change your mind—and you'll change your weight!

It's worth coming back to these restructured beliefs in the weeks ahead. It's even more important to learn to use this technique of "restructuring" yourself.

Here's an example.

Let's say you've been on the diet for six weeks. You're pleased with yourself, you feel you've learnt a lot, and you've certainly lost a really worthwhile amount of weight—even though you still have a fair way to go. Then you meet an old school friend, and she comments that you've really put on weight since she last saw you!

There are slimmers who would feel crushed and depressed—who would say to themselves: "What's the use? Everyone thinks I'm fat. I'll never change. It's hopeless. I'm just a fatty".

Fortunately, you won't be in that category! That was a typical example of the sort of twisted thinking that leads to negative thoughts and failure. One single incident was blown out of all proportion.

FACT 1: Everyone **doesn't** think you're fat. In fact, only one person mentioned it, and she wasn't in the position to see you have actually lost weight.

FACT 2: To say: "I'll never change" is absurd. You already have!

In other words, a single setback was generalised into a quite untrue perspective of failure—setting up a self-fulfilling prophecy.

FACT 3: You're not a "fatty"—you're a slim person in transition. This sort of "negative" labelling is very insidious, because putting yourself or other people in categories implies that they won't change. They do. Indeed, the same boss you may see as very authoritarian at work may be playful at home with her children.

Here is how you might now restructure your thoughts about the incident:

New belief: "My friend is quite entitled to notice that I've changed since we last met—in fact, it's just as well that I'm well on the way to regaining my old figure. I obviously acted just in time!

"I'll explain this exciting new Mind & Body approach to her, and give her some examples of what I've already learned. Maybe some other friends of hers could benefit."

See how the new way of looking at the incident can now be seen as a positive reinforcement of your success, not a threat to it?

So whenever you catch yourself saying or thinking something that doesn't support your new, positive expectation of success, look for other ways to express yourself, for other ways of looking at the situation. It is one of the most important factors in learning the skill to be slim.

THE BIG SECRET!

We've talked throughout this book about "mood" food—about how certain moods seem to trigger unnecessary eating. What we didn't ask was the vital question: "What triggers the mood in the first place?" If we could pinpoint that, we might prevent the mood from taking hold. Then you've really solved it—because you might never even want to get out the biscuit tin!

The big secret is that a mood doesn't just happen—something causes it. That something is **always** a thought. It cannot be any other way.

In the example we just saw, a depressed mood might easily have been triggered by the comment made by the friend that "you've put on weight". That then would have produced a series of negative thoughts.

However, in our example it didn't. Why?

Because we **stopped.** We **analysed** the sequence of thoughts and **put them in true perspective.** We decided that the reaction was:

1. Ridiculously generalised (e.g. "I'll never . . .")
2. All or nothing thinking (e.g. "Everyone thinks . . .")
3. Exaggerated thinking (e.g. "It's hopeless . . .")
4. Jumping to unwarranted conclusions (e.g. "What's the use?")
5. Negative labelling (e.g. "I'm just a fatty").

Let me make you a prediction. This type of twisted and negative thinking almost ALWAYS precedes a binge or a bout of unnecessary eating. BUT you can beat it with a *so* simple, but *so* powerful, technique.

STOP just before you begin to eat

ASK yourself what thought lead up to the mood and write down that sequence of thoughts (you'll be amazed at how accurately you remember).

It is absolutely vital, however, to **write down** the sequence, because your thoughts are so quick and slippery you can only pin them down if you write them down.

ANALYSE these thoughts for oversimplified, generalised, exaggerated and downright silly conclusions

Once you do that, you'll almost always see that your mood was not justified, because your thoughts were not well founded. And your urge to eat will disappear.

I've left this technique till last because I really believe it can be one of the most useful ideas, not just to enable you to be slim but to enable you to be in control of your whole life. Let's tackle real problems, not manufacture imaginary ones!

Now, however, the time has come to summarize everything we've learned.

> *"I think, therefore I am."*
> Descartes

WHAT WE LEARNED TOGETHER OVER THE LAST SIX WEEKS

More mind than body

* Successful slimming involves more "mind" than "body"! We are more psychological beings than logical ones.

* If you "used" food other than as nutrition, you need to find another way to handle that situation or problem.

  If it was resentment, remember forgiveness is a wonderfully selfish act!!

* There are two "yous"—the conscious and subconscious. They must both want the same thing!

* People talk of "trying" to diet, but the truth is that almost everyone has an inner resistance to losing weight. But you now understand the real situation, and how to reach the subconscious "you"—which is why, for the first time, you can succeed.

* The secret of successful slimming is not will power, it's imagination. You reach your imagination via your subconscious.

* The key to reaching your subconscious is strong, frequent visualisation of success. And frequent enthusiastic repetition of your affirmations.

  These condition your subconscious to want to produce a slim body. And your subconscious will find ways that will automatically bring about that desirable result.

* THINK slim and you will become slim.

* A positive self-approving frame of mind is essential. Look good and feel good about yourself.

* Act as if you have already successfully produced a more attractive physique. Having a regular hairdo, dressing well

and planning shopping trips for the clothes you will be able to wear, are all positive signals to the inner you that, this time, success is guaranteed.

* The power of a positive attitude is tremendous. A belief in your success becomes a self-fulfilling prophecy. The reverse is true too. I remember a friend who almost got to her target weight—after losing 60 lbs. I asked her what she was going to do with the clothes that were far too big. She said she'd keep them . . . just in case! Her mental image had not yet caught up with her slim new body. A case of a "fat head" still being on a slim body.

  However, by learning to physically enjoy her new slimness, and holding herself proudly, she was able to make the mental adjustment, too.

* You can change your actions and outlook incredibly quickly with the zoom technique. It's the most powerful way ever invented to put you in control of your mind—rather than having random, external events condition your mind and its beliefs.

* Your body's needs are important, too! Become aware of your body. Focus on whether you really want to eat. Use the concept of 1–5 eating. Listen to your body.

* Don't deny yourself your favourite foods. Instead, savour them. Create your own 6–10 scale of worthwhile foods.

* Become a Freedom (from Fat) Fighter.

* Incorporate high-nutrition/low-calorie foods into your everyday lifestyle. Don't count calories, but make every calorie count.

  If you cut down ruthlessly on fat, you need never bother about calorie counting.

* There seems to be a reluctance for people to tell the truth to people who are overweight.

  People who say: "You only need to eat sensibly" are missing a simple truth. If it was that easy, no one would have a problem.

We are all guilty of over-politeness. Someone says they should lose a little weight. Our reaction is: "No—you're fine". But we're doing them no favour.

* Successful slimmers share common characteristics with people who are successful in every other type of endeavour. They face facts!

And the facts are that:

1. Overweight is a health risk. If you are 20% over your ideal weight, you have an increased risk of:

   high blood pressure
   diabetes
   stroke
   heart attack
   gall stones
   varicose veins
   gout
   certain cancers
   reduced fertility

   That's why your commitment to the Mind & Body Programme should not just be for life—but to life.

2. Old-style dieting doesn't work. The average dieter tries 13 diets in his or her lifetime. Less than 10% succeed in keeping the weight off, because they haven't learnt the skill.

3 Exercise is important.

4. If you don't make changes, you will put unwanted fat back on.

* The Mind & Body Programme is a genuinely different approach. It's comprehensive and it deals with the mental changes that guarantee success this time. Incorporate the changes in your daily routine and you can forget dieting as an issue in your life for ever.

* Sometimes even small changes create a dramatically new result. They can turn a depressing negative into a total positive.

With two
small changes
IMPOSSIBLE
becomes
I'M POSSIBLE

That's what the Mind & Body Diet plan is—some small changes that can transform your attitude and life. Transform them into possibilities.

* The difference between people who keep the weight off, and those who don't, is purely one of attitude and motivation.
* They are the ones for whom the experience of a slim, energetic body is more pleasurable than the experience of overeating.
* They are the ones for whom the commitment to actually operate the 6–10 Food Scale and the 1–5 Eating Scale is worth making.
* They are the ones who put into practice the breathing and relaxation exercises.
* They are the ones who fill out the weekly Feedback Chart AND CONTINUE TO DO SO FOR AT LEAST ANOTHER SIX WEEKS.
* They are the ones who do exercise three times a week.
* They are the ones who use the "ZOOM" technique to manipulate their images to control their subconscious.
* They are the ones who do incorporate low-calorie/high-nutrition foods into their lifestyle.
* They are the ones who do create new perspectives on old and incorrect beliefs. Who turn negatives into positives. For them, a problem becomes a challenge.
* They are the ones who participate.

The choice is always yours.

DID YOU PARTICIPATE? – OR SPECTATE?

1. Your lifestyle questionnaire

At the beginning of Week One you filled out a private questionnaire. I have reproduced that questionnaire again. Please answer the same questions, using the same scale. When you have completed it, compare it with your answers in Week One. What differences do you notice?

I'm sure you will be pleasantly surprised at how much more positive your outlook is, and how much more control you have over your eating—and, I suspect, your life generally.

2. Your goal weight

Six weeks ago you filled out your lbs lost goal and target weight. How have you fared?

Do you still have weight to lose? In which case, set a new target and go for it!

The reason I propose you set another six-week target is because it's a time scale that everyone can visualise and there's a great sense of success in achieving these six-week goals—even if six weeks alone does not achieve your ultimate target. If you've got a big task to achieve, it's easier to break it down into bite-size pieces.

There's an old phrase that queries: "How do you eat an elephant?" The answer is: "One bite at a time!"

3. Lara's theme

We know that LEARNING is all about AWARENESS, REVIEW and ACTION.

Awareness

I think the two most important elements in being aware are the Hunger-Meter and the Food-o-Meter. In other words, sticking to 1–5 eating and choosing 6–10 foods. Trusting your body. Have you incorporated them into your lifestyle?

There's no better way of getting in touch with your body.

Review

Did you keep a weekly feedback chart? It's the best way of judging how far you have managed to incorporate the changes we know work. Reread the charts and draw your own conclusions on them.

Action

* Did you use the stickers? On your fridge? On your larder door? In the kitchen?
* Did you exercise?
* Did you follow the Ten Commandments of the Freedom (from Fat) Fighter?
* Have you incorporated three deep breathing and relaxation moments of peace into your day?
* Are you using the "ZOOM" technique to change your response to situations or moods that previously triggered unnecessary eating?

This is understandably the most 'unfamiliar' action I have requested you to make. But I also know it's the most powerful. If you don't use the "ZOOM" technique, you are ignoring one of the most useful techniques available to you.

And why would you ignore it? Because it's strange? Because it's manipulating your own mind?

If that's the reason, you are effectively saying that you are happy for your previous experience, for other people, and for random past events, to be the factors that create your attitudes and beliefs. That you would rather be controlled than do the controlling. I doubt if that's what you really want. Try it!

A FINAL THOUGHT

I remember vividly an incident from my childhood. Some friends and I were playing near a stream on a sunny day.

There were grassy banks on either side and a fallen, quite narrow, tree trunk spanned the stream. The tree trunk wasn't all that long—perhaps 12 feet. The drop to the stream wasn't all that high—perhaps 5 feet. And the stream certainly wasn't deep. Yet we were all frightened to make our way across the tree trunk because, of course, we feared we might overbalance and fall in. The more we hesitated, the more nervous we felt.

Suddenly I decided to just do it. The action banished the fear. I was over in a second and, within moments, so were my friends.

Clearly, this was a very trivial event, but it made a deep impression on me.

There are times in our lives when the only thing to do is to take action, and that single decisive moment conquers all.

YOU CAN'T WIN IF YOU DON'T BEGIN.

Have you begun to incorporate all these thoughts and recommendations into your lifestyle?

YOUR LIFESTYLE QUESTIONNAIRE – SIX WEEKS LATER

Name	**Age**	**Height weight**	**Current goal weight**

Answer the questions below, using the 'scale' provided. Ring the number that most nearly expresses your situation.

Question	1	2	3	4	5	6	7
1. When did you first have a weight problem?	Age?		Reason?				
2. When you start to eat do you usually feel:	1 Already full	2	3	4 Comfortable	5	6	7 Hungry
3. When you stop eating are you usually:	1 Stuffed full	2	3	4 Satisfied - just right	5	6	7 Still hungry
4. Do you eat between meals?	1 Often	2	3	4	5	6	7 Never
5. How often are you dieting?	1 Always	2	3	4 Sometimes	5	6	7 Never
6. How often do you eat foods you absolutely love?	1 Never	2	3	4	5	6	7 Always
7. Do you like your body?	1 No	2	3	4	5	6	7 Yes
8. Do you feel controlled by food?	1 No	2	3	4	5	6	7 Yes
9. Do you ever visualise yourself being slim?	1 Never	2	3	4	5	6	7 Always
10. Do you feel guilty about eating?	1 Yes, very	2	3	4	5	6	7 No
11. Do you eat when you're stressed or bored?	1 Often	2	3	4	5	6	7 Never
12. Do you eat when you are worried or unhappy?	1 Often	2	3	4	5	6	7 Never
13. How often do you have a good binge?	1 Often	2	3	4	5	6	7 Never
14. How is your self-esteem?	1 Low	2	3	4	5	6	7 High
15. Do you look forward to eating alone?	1 Often	2	3	4	5	6	7 Rarely

Finally, mark your own life on a 1 to 7 scale (1 meaning poor, 7 meaning excellent) for the following factors.

I rate these areas of my life as follows, on a 1–7 scale.
1 would be low, 7 would be excellent.

Job satisfaction	1	2	3	4	5	6	7
Exercise level	1	2	3	4	5	6	7
Energy level	1	2	3	4	5	6	7
Family relationships	1	2	3	4	5	6	7
Health	1	2	3	4	5	6	7
Sex life	1	2	3	4	5	6	7
Stress (1 high/7 low)	1	2	3	4	5	6	7
Friendships	1	2	3	4	5	6	7

N.B. Do you notice how much your rating of your life has improved? How your satisfaction with yourself and your life has increased? How many more high scores you can now ring?

The truth is that the skills of being slim are similar to the skills you need in most aspects of life.

THE MIND & BODY DIET™

What do you **really** need to know about nutrition?

NUTRITION – WHAT DO YOU REALLY NEED TO KNOW?

There are six types of nutrients—carbohydrates, protein, fat, vitamins, minerals and water. Only the first three have calories.

Carbohydrates

They're made up of carbon, oxygen and hydrogen (hence the name carb-o-hydrate!) Ultimately, every single form gets broken down in your body into the type of sugar you use for energy—glucose.

Your blood only carries a few minutes' supply of glucose at any one time, but your brain and muscles need a constant source so your liver needs to work steadily to produce it. Even your liver doesn't store more than about 12 hours' supply, which is why a breakfast (literally break-the-fast) is important and should contain carbohydrate.

Some carbohydrate is complex—which means it's made up of lots of different sugars bound together. These carbohydrates are fruit, bread, cereals, pasta, vegetables and rice.

Other carbohydrates are simple—like honey and sugar (sucrose). The body absorbs them quickest but they have almost no nutritional value. Moreover, refined sugars are easy to eat in large amounts because they pack in a lot of calories per ounce. In contrast, complex carbohydrates are much bulkier and so you have far less calories per ounce. So you can fill up without taking in so many calories.

Carbohydrates are the body's basic and most efficient source of energy and fuel.

Protein

As we all know, protein is the stuff that builds the tissue in our bodies. It contains 22 amino acids that eventually combine in various ways to form our hair, skin, muscles, organs, etc.

Protein can also be broken down in the body to glucose and used as energy, but neither carbohydrate nor fat can be converted to protein. Consequently, you need a minimum amount of protein every day.

Of the 22 amino acids, the body itself can make 13, but only your food can provide the other nine. So these are called the essential amino acids.

You can either get these nine essential amino acids by eating a combination of foods—for example, combining beans + wheat or cereals + leafy vegetables or bread + cheese—or you can get them by eating animal protein, because the animal has already done the job for you!

A woman needs about 40–55 grams of protein a day, a man from 50–70 grams.

Fat

Dietary fat contains several fatty acids. The body can manufacture all but two of these fatty acids. Consequently, these are called essential fatty acids. They are linoleic and linolenic acid.

Dietary fat also ensures that we can absorb the vital vitamins that are stored in fat—namely Vitamins A, D, E and K. So we do need fat—but not nearly as much as we eat!

You will naturally be aware of the difference between saturated fat and polyunsaturated fat. There is in fact a third form—monounsaturated fat—the type you find in olive oil.

Excess of all three types of fat is bad for you, but in addition you should make a conscious attempt to significantly reduce the saturated fats in your diet. They are the ones that are solid at room temperature and are found in animal fat, coconut fat, cocoa butter and palm oil.

Watch, too, for processed foods that are labelled hydrogenated. The manufacturer of, for example, hydrogenated margarine has—in his wisdom (!)—taken polyunsaturated oil and, by treating it with hydrogen, has produced a form of fat that's just as bad for you as saturated fat. Saturated fat is the form that's linked strongly to heart disease and cancer.

Vitamins

Essentially, vitamins are chemicals that help you process the other nutrients, and they promote a wide range of chemical reactions in your body. There are 13 vitamins.

For example:

* The B vitamins help break down sugars into energy.
* Vitamin A is needed for healthy skin, eyes and digestion.
* Vitamin B_2 helps the body use oxygen efficiently.
* Vitamin B_{12} is essential for the nervous system.
* Folic acid is essential for the production of red blood cells and the nervous system.
* Vitamin C is needed for healthy tissue.
* Vitamin K helps prevent fatty acids from oxidising in the blood.

And so on.

The point is not to memorise what vitamins do, but to eat correctly to get them all.

I'll tell you how shortly.

Minerals

There are 21 essential minerals. Some are produced from gases and you need them in large quantities, like hydrogen, carbon, oxygen and nitrogen. Some you need in small quantities, like calcium, potassium, magnesium and sodium.

Some others you need in minute quantities, like nickel, iron, copper, manganese, molybdenum and selenium. We call these trace elements, but they are also essential.

You need minerals because they enable electrical activity to take place in your body. (The "spark" of life is, essentially, literally true). Minerals also help store and distribute water and help to facilitate the chemical reactions that take place in your body and brain every minute of every day. They also regulate muscle constriction.

Again, you'd be wasting your time if you tried to remember what each mineral does. Just learn to get enough, but not too much!

Water

You can live for up to 50 days without food. You'd die in 5 without water. On a hot day, it could be 24 hours!

Every day you lose about 5 pints of water—3 you excrete, 2 you lose in perspiration and exhalation from your lungs.

That's why you need so much!

Balance

There are 45 nutrients in all and they all work together. To say that a particular vitamin will clear up your health problems is like saying that a symphony would sound better played on a tuba!

To make beautiful music needs a full complement of instruments working together in harmony.

To be healthy needs all the nutrients in the correct balance—again, working harmoniously together. That means eating a wide enough range of foods to ensure that you get all the vitamins and minerals—but at the same time ensuring that you don't get an excess of any individual one. Much like a conductor ensures that no one instrument drowns out the rest.

Most dietitians put food into 4 groups. If you eat from each group each day, you'll get a reasonable balance.

The groups are:-

(1)
Meat
Fish
Poultry
Eggs
Cheese
Nuts
Pulses

This is the protein group and a source of Vitamins B_{12}, A and D.

(2)
Grains
Bread
Cereals
Pasta
Carrots
Starchy vegetables
(corn, potatoes)

This group is an excellent source of energy from complex carbohydrate plus, especially, the B vitamins, Vitamin E iron and fibre.

(3)
Leafy vegetables
Fruits
Tomatoes

Excellent sources of Vitamins A, B_1, B_2, Niacin folic acid, Vitamin C, iron, magnesium and potassium.

(4)
Milk
Yoghurt
Cheese

This group provides protein, calcium, Vitamins A, B_1, B_{12} and D.

There are other food groups—fats, alcohol and sugar—but the problem is not to eat enough of these—it's to restrict our intake!

The title of this section is "What do you **really** need to know about nutrition?"

I think the simplest way to answer that question is to:

a. Eat from the 4 food groups daily.

b. Be aware of what you might be deficient in—and emphasise foods that supply these nutrients.

c. Be aware of what you might have in excess and eat to reduce these nutrients.

d. Be aware that there are some specialist nutrients that have specific health benefits.

NUTRIENTS THAT YOU MAY LACK

Folic Acid

This 'B' vitamin is essential for healthy blood formation, the proper working of the central nervous system and when cells are dividing quickly, e.g. during pregnancy.

It is also the most common deficiency. Some studies show over 90% of women lack proper intake of folic acid. Best food sources are liver, kidney, green vegetables, eggs, whole-grain cereals. Absorption is aided by Vitamin C.

Vitamin B_6

This vitamin is important for the metabolism of protein and the proper function of the nervous system. Deficiencies will show up in irritability, nervousness and sleep problems. Good sources are meats, fish, eggs, whole-grain cereals.

Calcium

Inadequate calcium can make you susceptible to osteoporosis —a weakening of bone structure that leads to breakages later in life. Get calcium from milk products, leafy vegetables, beans and nuts. A high-fat or high-protein diet can reduce your ability to absorb calcium. Vitamin D assists absorption.

Regular exercise also assists calcium absorption.

Iron

Women, especially, can very often be iron deficient. Since it helps in healthy blood formation, you'll feel tired if you are.

Iron-rich foods are liver, kidney, egg yolk, shellfish and legumes. Other less good sources are meats, fish, poultry and cereals.

Vitamin C improves the extent to which you absorb iron, but tea and coffee reduce your ability to absorb it.

Zinc

Zinc is fast becoming one of the most studied minerals. It is essential for full sexual maturation and a deficiency can cause hair loss, skin problems, an impaired sense of taste, impaired immune reaction, white spots on nails, and reduced ability to heal.

The refining of food substantially reduces its zinc content and high-protein and high-fibre diets also reduce the amount of zinc you absorb. People with a high alcohol intake are also frequently deficient.

The best dietary sources of zinc are steak, chops, liver, egg yolk, wholewheat and cereals, peas, nuts, chicken and shellfish.

THE NUTRIENTS YOU MAY WELL HAVE IN EXCESS

Sodium

The average person needs from 1.2 to 3 grams of sodium a day. We actually average about 6—about 300% too much!

It comes, of course, from the salt we add, from processed foods and from the natural salt in food. It's a potential hazard, as excess sodium is implicated strongly in high blood pressure.

The most practical way to reduce sodium is to use a salt substitute, because these use potassium to provide a "salty" taste and potassium can actually help lower blood pressure.

The other obvious action is to read labels and avoid food with more than 200mg of sodium per portion. Go easy on these high sodium foods. They are:-

- Bacon
- Green olives
- Ham
- Processed cheese
- Processed crisps and nuts
- Cornflakes
- Cheese biscuits
- Canned almonds
- Canned soups
- Soy sauce

The other excellent tip is to use lemon juice, herbs and spices as flavour-enhancers.

Sugar

We consume, as a nation, 5 times as much refined sugar as we did fifty years ago!

Apart from the obvious way to cut it down (eliminating it in tea and coffee) it's well worth while reading labels:

a. Go for fruit canned in juice—not syrup.

b. Be aware of manufacturers who list sucrose, fructose, honey and maltadextrine separately on their labels. They are **all** sugars!

c. Be aware that colas and soft drinks can contain up to 5 teaspoonfuls of sugar per can!

d. Cut down on sweets, desserts and cakes.

Now that you know how excess sugar intake can cause so many problems by overstimulating your insulin production, you would be very wise to substantially reduce your intake of this source of "empty calories".

Cholesterol

Whilst cholesterol is not a nutrient, it is necessary for the body's healthy function. Every cell in your body contains it. It is a waxy substance that is both produced by the body and eaten in food.

High levels of cholesterol in the blood are linked strongly to heart disease and strokes. What happens is that cholesterol deposits can start to build up on the walls of the arteries. This then makes it difficult for the arteries to expand and contract in response to changes in blood flow as your heart beats. If the arteries narrow too much, the flow of blood can stop and the cells beyond the stoppage die.

If the stoppage happens in an artery leading to the heart, you suffer a coronary attack. If it occurs in an artery leading to the brain, it's a stroke.

Neither of these occurrences is a happy prospect. So what should you do?

a. Check your cholesterol level through your doctor.

b. Increase your intake of soluble fibre.

c. Seriously consider the benefits of the Omega 3 supplement that we will shortly discuss.

d. Reduce your intake of saturated fats. They're the fats in beef, lamb, pork, ham, cream, cheese and butter. Also the fats in coconut oil, palm oil and cocoa butter.

Remember, hydrogenated fats are just as undesirable.

e. Reducing saturated fat is, interestingly, even more vital than reducing the amount of cholesterol in the food—though this, too, is important.

Food	**Quantity**	**Mg of cholesterol**
Chicken liver	4 oz	846
Calves liver (fried)	4 oz	500
Scrambled egg	2 oz	263
Poached egg	One	242
Shrimp	4 oz	170
Butter	2 oz	132
Roast turkey (dark)	4 oz	115
Hamburger	4 oz	107
Fried chicken	4 oz	102
Cream	2 oz	80
Cheddar cheese	4 oz	112
Cottage cheese	4 oz	6

The basic rule of thumb is to limit your dietary cholesterol to about 400mg a day.

DO I NEED ANY NUTRITIONAL SUPPLEMENTS?

It's difficult to say.

If you are eating from the four food groups, and are using one of the Uni-Vite food range each day as part of a general plan to increase your intake of high-nutrition/low-calorie foods, you would be unlikely to need any further supplement—because each Uni-Vite meal contains 1/3 of your daily requirement of every single essential nutrient.

There are, however, three forms of supplement we do recommend. Each one is for a specific group of people.

Food Tabs

Two categories of people may generally have increased nutrient needs. Teenagers and the elderly.

Teenagers because they do have extra nutritional demands during this important period of growth, and because they are notorious for eating junk food. The elderly because they often do not eat enough to obtain an adequate level of all the nutrients.

For both groups, Uni-Vite have produced a real food solution— a product called "Food Tabs". Food Tabs consist of a tasty, crunchy, chocolate snack, each snack containing one quarter of a day's principal vitamins and minerals in just 19 calories. In fact, each Food Tab contains somewhat more of the key nutrients iron, folic acid and Vitamin C (about 1/3 of a day's allowance).

So two Food Tabs a day provide at least half the average person's basic vitamins and minerals.

G.L.A.

Polyunsaturated fat is a normal component of our everyday food diet, of course. Most people can metabolise polyunsaturated fat into an essential form of fatty acid called G.L.A. (Gamma Linolenic Acid). In turn G.L.A. regulates some vital hormonal activities.

In some people, however, this natural process is impaired. They cannot produce enough G.L.A., so their hormonal activity does not operate properly.

For them, it becomes desirable to take G.L.A. in a "ready made" form. The beneficial results are dramatic. Twenty-three out of Britain's thirty medical schools are researching the benefits of G.L.A. for people suffering from pre-menstrual tension, rheumatoid arthritis, skin problems and diabetes. Until now the main source of G.L.A. has been Evening Primrose Oil. Now, however, a purer, double-strength form of G.L.A. is available— which Uni-Vite market quite simple as G.L.A.

G.L.A. can often bring about very quick and measurable relief in cases of PMT, skin complaints and in helping to alleviate the symptoms of arthritis.

Omega 3

Some years ago, scientists began to investigate why it is that Eskimoes, who eat a very high-fat diet, have such a low incidence of heart disease. It should have been the reverse.

The answer lay in the fact that they eat a diet very high in fish—particularly "oily" fish like salmon, herring and mackerel. And a nutrient in this fish oil, called Omega 3, helps lower the level of cholesterol in the blood, and reduces the blood's tendency to clot, which in turn lowers the risk of heart disease.

The British Medical Journal reported recently that the nutrients in Omega 3 are "the most potent inhibitors of thrombosis found in ordinary diets". In plain English, Omega 3 helps prevent heart disease.

The problem is that the average British diet is low in this nutrient—unless you have an exceptionally high intake of mackerel, herring, sardines and salmon.

Omega 3 supplements are available—and again, Uni-Vite markets its product under the simple name "Omega 3".

The relative contribution of Omega 3 per 4 oz serving by type of fish is:

Sardines (oil-packed)	5.5 grams
Sardines (water-packed)	4.5 grams
King salmon	3.6 grams
Tuna	2.5 grams
Mackerel	2.2 grams
Herring	Av. 2.0 grams
Trout	1.0 grams
White fish	Av. 0.3 grams

So what's the final answer to the question: "Do I need any nutritional supplements?"

I think a fair reply would be:

* If you are an adult and you eat according to the advice in the Mind and Body Programme, the answer is probably: "No".

* If you do take a vitamin-mineral pill, make sure it only provides 100% maximum of the Recommended Daily Amounts (R.D.A.s). Many store brands do.,

  Food Tabs have been designed to let you achieve anything from a 25% to a 100% supplement. I'd recommend them, or a store vitamin/mineral supplement, to the elderly—and to many teenagers.

* The effect of a G.L.A. supplement can be remarkable and noticed within one month. If you have any of the problems mentioned above, it is worth trying, and it's perfectly safe.

* People with a high heart disease and stroke risk should seriously consider taking Omega 3 regularly. It, again, is safe, and since heart disease is the U.K.'s No. 1 killer, many could benefit.

FINAL THOUGHT

Nutrition is a fascinating and fast-developing science. No area is more fascinating than medical studies currently in progress that show that many of the modern degenerative diseases are linked to the reaction of oxygen and fat in our bloodstream.

This reaction releases some very damaging chemicals called "free radicals". And free radicals can trigger body changes that, in turn, can lead to cancer, heart disease, strokes and arthritis.

The above research makes it clear that, if we can reduce the damaging effect of free radicals, we may well be able to reduce the risk of some of our most serious diseases. The key seems to be to reduce the degree to which oxygen and fat react in our bodies. And the key to that, in turn, is likely to be nutrition.

Some nutrients have the specific effect of reducing the damaging internal oxidisation of fat. They are the anti-oxidant nutrients that include Vitamin E, Vitamin A, Vitamin C, selenium, chromium, zinc and some amino acids.

Uni-Vite is involved in this research.

THE MIND & BODY DIET™

Your questions answered

THE UNI-VITE DIET FOODS

Why is Uni-Vite a personalised diet?

Because the calorie and protein needs of a 6'0" man and a 5'2" woman are obviously different.

The UK Department of Health has produced a report recommending that:

Women up to 5'8" should not employ a diet that contains below 400 calories a day and 40g protein.

Men (and women of 5'8" and over) should not use any diet below 500 calories a day and 50g of protein.

The Uni-Vite Diet Programme recommends daily intakes that are above these minimums and does differentiate between the nutritional needs of men and women.

The other obvious reason is that each individual's tastes and circumstances are different. Some people have a very low metabolic rate and need the lowest calorie intake compatible with safety to be able to lose weight at a satisfying rate.

Other people—usually men—can sustain a steady weight loss of 4 lbs a week at 600, 700 or even 800 calories a day.

By offering a really good range of hot foods, soups, drinks and bars in plenty of flavours, there is enough variety to ensure that you enjoy your food, yet lose weight continuously.

And because every single Uni-Vite meal contains 1/3 of your daily requirement of vitamins, minerals and trace elements, you can mix and match any three of the meals to achieve your ideal calorie level and still be assured of complete nutrition.

Is Uni-Vite a Very Low Calorie diet?

No. The whole point of a personalised diet is that it ensures that the calorie and protein level is appropriate for your sex, age, height and exercise level.

The average person would therefore use a Uni-Vite diet plan of 600 calories a day or more. Below that, the UK Department of Health defines diets as Very Low Calorie.

It is, of course, possible that a below-average person (in terms of nutritional needs) will require a below-average diet. Thus an older woman of below average height, and below average activity, might need a calorie level of 450 calories a day in order to achieve a satisfactory rate of weight loss.

In which case the specific permission of the doctor is required.

I've read that you can lose muscle on diets below 1000 calories, and that's dangerous

The easy answer is that the Uni-Vite programme is very definitely safe. A whole series of clinical trials have been conducted. They all show that weight loss is encouraging—an average of 16 lbs a month—and that all important muscle tissue is maintained. Indeed, Dr Alfred Wirth, an eminent cardiologist, says that "cardiac (heart) function is actually improved on the Uni-Vite programme."

What you **will** lose on any diet is body protein. You see, when you put on weight, you put it on in the ratio of about 70% extra fat and 30% extra protein. This protein includes a larger skin area, more blood volume, extra fat cell structure, and larger muscles in, especially, the legs.

When you lose weight, protein is, of course, lost from exactly the same sources. The important fact is to know that this protein is lost in a similar proportion to that in which it is gained.

In a fully-supervised long-term study at St Mary's Hospital, London, a Uni-Vite consultant, Dr Victor Wynn, Professor of Metabolism, found that on a 600 calorie diet, 93% of weight loss was fat and only 7% was protein. Proof positive that the Uni-Vite programme is safe and promotes what you want—fat loss.

I've read of the Cambridge Diet—is Uni-Vite the same?

No. The Cambridge Diet is classified as a Very Low Calorie Diet and was introduced as a 330 calorie a day diet for both men and women, although it has now been modified to 405 calories.

What are the long-term effects of the Uni-Vite Personalised Diet?

Uni-Vite has, through the University of Surrey, carried out studies on users 1 year, 2 years and even 3 years after they initially used the product.

The key results of the 1 year follow-up study in 1985 were:

> 94% had tried to lose weight before
>
> 84% found it easier with the Uni-Vite Plan
>
> 71% of users' doctors actively encouraged them to follow the Uni-Vite Plan
>
> 71% of Uni-Vite dieters noticed a specific improvement in their health.
>
> 87% found it easier to maintain their weight with the plan.
>
> 77% said the role of the Advisor was important.

What medical benefits can be expected from a successful weight loss on Uni-Vite?

Clinical tests show that significant reductions in blood pressure can be achieved, along with reductions of cholesterol and triglycerides (i.e. fat) in the blood.

Do I need to check with my doctor?

Experts recommend that you consult your doctor before any weight loss programme.

Certainly, if your personalised programme indicates a sole source plan with a calorie level below 600 calories a day, you must check with your physician before starting the plan.

Is the Uni-Vite Low Calorie Programme suitable for everyone?

There are some people who should not be on any diet.

* Pregnant or lactating women, for example, unless they are under strict medical supervision.
* People who have suffered a stroke or heart attack, or with kidney disease.
* People undergoing steroid therapy.
* Hypoglycaemiacs.

Additionally, no teenager under 17 should use the programme unless their doctor approves, and diabetics must also consult their physician. Although for Type II diabetics the Uni-Vite Programme may well be an ideal way to reduce medication, only your doctor can advise.

Why does the Uni-Vite Plan recommend drinking so much water?

Our bodies consist of over 60% water. Also, when the body loses fat, it also loses water. So we need to constantly replace our body fluids and also to keep our kidneys functioning properly.

Dieters also find that sodium (salt) can build up in their kidneys causing water retention—often the cause of an apparent weight "plateau". Drinking plenty of water can, ironically, help prevent this fluid retention.

Can I drink alcohol on the diet?

No. Your body, on the diet, is receiving high-grade nutrition in less than normal bulk. If you drink alcohol, it will affect you fast!

Moreover, alcohol is not only fattening in itself—ounce for ounce, almost twice as fattening as protein or carbohydrate— but is usually associated in our minds with snacking and high calorie meals.

If I lose weight quickly, will I get gaunt?

No. The most common comments from Uni-Vite slimmers are how energetic they feel, how their nails and hair seem to grow faster, how much their skin glows and how firm it is.

Since Uni-Vite contains every single nutrient (over 45 in every meal) you can get perfectly balanced nutrition each time. The only thing you deprive yourself of is calories!

How much weight can I lose?

How much do you want to lose? Uni-Vite slimmers have lost 10 stone or more. About one stone, or 14 lbs, a month seems to be the average.

Will I be hungry if I stick to just three Uni-Vite meals a day?

After the first two days, few people are hungry. And even during the first two days, it's rarely physical hunger—it's more that you expect you must surely be hungry on a low-calorie level!

Does Uni-Vite contain any preservatives?

No. It's natural food—free of all preservatives, drugs, diuretics or artificial colouring.

Are there any side-effects?

About 8% of Uni-Vite dieters experience some side-effects while they adjust to what is, after all, a deliberately major change from their usual eating patterns.

These can include a headache—often due to less caffeine. Drinking plenty of water is the answer.

It may also include slight dizziness when you stand up quickly. That's because losing fat quickly has a diuretic effect, which reduces the fluid in your stomach. Drink plenty of water!

What about fibre?

We're fibre fans in an ongoing diet—as you've seen. And there's a good level of fibre in the "Whole Meals" and the "Micro Bars". Nonetheless, whilst you are on the Uni-Vite Diet Programme itself, which is low bulk, there's no evidence you need much fibre.

I'm confused! What's the difference between a formula diet, a fad diet, a crash diet and a calorie-reduced diet?

* *Formula diets,* like the Uni-Vite Plan, are nutritionally complete, balanced meals delivering all 45+ nutrients that the body requires. To provide these nutrients, food technologists take natural food sources such as milk, eggs and soya, remove any parts that are surplus to requirements (such as fat), and fortify them with vitamins, minerals and trace elements to ensure 100% nutrition. The result is complete nutrition in 25% of normal calories.

* *A fad diet* is a diet which will claim a quick weight loss but is nutritionally deficient and potentially damaging to your health. Fad diets often sound more appealing than "sensible" reducing diets but their chances of long-term success are virtually nil.

* *A crash diet* is a starvation diet where you simply reduce your food intake, again with no regard to balanced nutrition. Starvation diets tend to burn muscle tissue as well as adipose fat (the non-essential fat that we want to lose), which results in a drawn or haggard look. Again, the chances of long-term success are slim

and, in fact, there is a tendency to increase weight more rapidly once you start eating again, because your body has gone into a defensive mode and severely reduced your metabolic rate in order to retain your energy stores.

* *A calorie-reduced diet* is a diet which is nutritionally balanced using ordinary foods, but tends to be slow and boring with excessive weighing and measuring of portions and many "forbidden" foods.

Achieving your target weight is possible by any of the dietary methods mentioned above but, human nature being what it is, we need quick results for encouragement, as long as the method we are using is safe.

The fad and the crash diets are obviously dangerous and should be avoided, although it is probable that many dieters have tried them.

The calorie-reduced diet can work but tends to be slow, requires a lot of will power, effort and disruption and, in fact, has a poor record of long-term success.

Isn't a formula diet an expensive way to slim?

Actually, it's a cheap way to slim!

If you use the Uni-Vite range as your **sole** source of nutrition, you'd currently expect it to cost an average of about £13.00 a week.

The average expenditure on food in the UK was £14.39 a week in October 1988. Organisations such as Weight Watchers do a good job—but you pay a weekly registration fee of about £3 whether you attend or not. Of course, you still buy your regular £14.39 worth of food in addition.

Diet centres offer a similar service to the Uni-Vite Mind and Body Programme, i.e. provide food plus advice and support. However, a typical weekly cost would be £35.00.

So the Uni-Vite Diet is actually the least expensive way to slim.

Won't I be tired on a low-calorie diet?

No. The almost universal comment that Uni-Vite slimmers make is that they feel so well and energetic.

You see, you will still get all the energy you need, even if you are taking in only 600 calories a day. The Uni-Vite foods provide 600 of these calorie needs. The remaining calories are taken from your unwanted fat stores—which is exactly what you want!

CALCULATING YOUR GOAL WEIGHT

There are several tables of ideal weight. The latest method, recommended by nutritionists, is the Body Mass Index, or B.M.I. It's actually calculated by dividing your weight, in kilos, by your height in metres. Since few of us, however, have a PhD in Mathematics, we've worked it out for you!

The idea is that there is an upper and a lower limit to your ideal B.M.I. from 21 to 25. Of course, this is for both men and women, so generally a woman's ideal weight will tend to be towards the lower end of the two limits below.

Use the table as a guide to set your ideal weight.

	Your weight should be between:	
If your height is:	**Lower limit: B.M.I. = 21**	**Upper limit: B.M.I. = 25**
5' 0"	7st 5lbs	8st 11lbs
5' 1"	7st 12lbs	9st 6lbs
5' 2"	8st 2lbs	9st 10lbs
5' 3"	8st 7lbs	10st 1lbs
5' 4"	8st 10lbs	10st 5lbs
5' 5"	8st 13lbs	10st 10lbs
5' 6"	9st 4lbs	11st 0lbs
5' 7"	9st 8lbs	11st 4lbs
5' 8"	9st 13lbs	11st 11lbs
5' 9"	10st 1lbs	12st 1lbs
5' 10"	10st 5lbs	12st 6lbs
5' 11"	10st 10lbs	12st 10lbs
6' 0"	11st 0lbs	13st 1lb
6' 1"	11st 4lbs	13st 7lbs
6' 2"	11st 9lbs	13st 12lbs

N.B. 14 lbs = 1 stone

Deciding on your personal daily calorie level

Use the simple checklist below. Tick the box on each line that applies to you. Then add up the points. The total will give you a daily calorie level on the Uni-Vite diet that's appropriate for you personally.

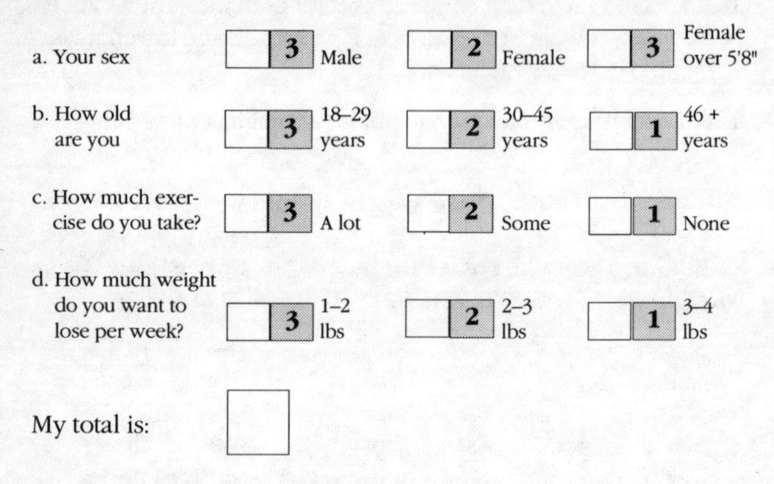

a. Your sex	3 Male	2 Female	3 Female over 5'8"
b. How old are you	3 18–29 years	2 30–45 years	1 46 + years
c. How much exercise do you take?	3 A lot	2 Some	1 None
d. How much weight do you want to lose per week?	3 1–2 lbs	2 2–3 lbs	1 3–4 lbs

My total is:

Example: An average-height woman of 35 who takes NO exercise and who wants to lose weight quickly—i.e. 3 to 4 lbs a week—would score 6. A 26 year old man who exercises moderately and wants to lose 4 lbs a week or more would score 9.

Having determined your points total, now refer to the following simple table. It tells you the number of daily calories that is appropriate for your sex, age, exercise level and desired speed of weight loss.

If your score was	This is the number of calories you need per day on the Uni-Vite Diet
5	500*
6	600
7	600–700
8	700–800
9	800
10 or over	900

*specifically requires doctor's approval

Now all that remains to do is to choose a combination of Uni-Vite low-calorie/high-nutrition foods that provide your personal daily calorie level.

Uni-Vite, or your Advisor, will help you to do that when you telephone or write in, but the range is listed below to guide you.

There is only one more IMPORTANT point to notice. A recent government report (C.O.M.A.) recommended that the MINIMUM number of calories for any woman on a formula diet should be 400 per day, providing 40 grams of protein. The minimum number of calories for any man on a formula diet should be 500 calories per day, providing 50 grams of protein.

Moreover, if you go this low in calories, you should not be on a formula diet as a sole source of nutrition for more than 3–4 weeks.

Our experience with the Uni-Vite Programme, on a worldwide basis and involving over 3 million slimmers, is that a wiser MINIMUM for women is 500 calories a day and for men is 600 calories a day.

Sticking to a 600 calorie diet will give you all the speed of weight loss you could possibly want and (subject to your doctor's permission if total intake is below 600) you can safely continue to follow such a programme until you do reach your target weight.

It is far better to achieve your goal by following a fast, steady, **continuous** slimming regime than to have to diet in short bursts using a **very** low calorie diet.

How much can you lose in six weeks?

A realistic target for women would be 14–24 lbs. A realistic target for men would be 18–30 lbs.

The more weight you have to lose, the higher will be your rate of weight loss. The average weight loss achieved on our trials was 20 lbs for women, 27 lbs for men over a six week period.

Choosing your Uni-Vite foods

Before you go on the diet, you should request either from the Uni-Vite company or from your Advisor the brochure on the diet. Read it carefully and you will be fully informed. You can, of course, show it to your doctor—who should be consulted before you go on this or any other diet.

However, to guide you, the list opposite indicates the current range of foods that is available to be "mixed and matched" to create a diet that's nutritionally ideal for you personally, and which suits your own tastes.

You will see that ANY three meals provide 100% of your vitamin and mineral needs and 100% of a woman's protein needs. However, should any three of these meals, soups or drinks fail to reach the calorie or protein level you have set yourself, then a 10 oz glass of skimmed milk will contribute approximately 90 calories and 10 grams of protein to your daily total and should normally be all you ever need to add.

The big advantage of the Uni-Vite diet is that everything is so blissfully simple. There are no calories to count, no portions to weigh or complicated menus to prepare. Just add hot or cold water to the sachet,, as appropriate, and you have a meal.

Suggested meal occasion	Product	Calories per serving	% of Vitamin and Mineral needs per serving	Protein per serving	Flavours available	Contains fibre?
Breakfast	*Micro Muesli*	*250*	*33%*	*15g*	*Natural*	*Yes*
Lunch	*Micro Soups*	*110*	*33%*	*14g*	*Chicken* *Vegetable* *Turkey*	—
Lunch	*Micro Bars*	*250*	*33%*	*15g*	*Peanut* *Orange* *Cinnamon*	*Yes*
Dinner	*Whole Meals*	*205*	*33%*	*15g*	*Chilli* *Curry* *Pasta*	*Yes*
Any time	*Micro Drinks*	*110*	*33%*	*14g*	*Chocolate* *Strawberry* *Vanilla* *Coffee* *Banana* *Butterscotch*	—
Any time	*Uni-Vite Gold Drinks & Soups* *(These are richer, thicker and contain 60% more protein)*	*210*	*33%*	*23g*	*Chocolate* *Vanilla* *Vegetable Soup*	—

The address of Uni-Vite for enquiries, or to find your nearest Advisor, or to order on a post-free basis (48 hour delivery) is:

Uni-Vite Ltd
Uni-Vite House
50 Aylesbury Road
Aston Clinton
Aylesbury
Bucks HP22 5AH

Telephone: (0296) 631177
Fax: (0296) 631074

In New Zealand, contact Uni-Vite NZ Ltd, 2 Expo Place, PO Box 24123, Christchurch. Telephone (3) 844072.

In Canada, contact Uni-Vite Nutrition Inc, 50 Paxman Road, Unit 12a & 14, Etobicoke, Ontario, M9C 1B6.

In Australia, contact Uni-Vite Nutrition Pty Ltd, PO Box 424, Greensborough 3088.

Team Trim Groups

The above addresses can be contacted if you wish to form a slimming group with your friends.

Beyond Week Six

For those of you who have particularly enjoyed delving into the mind of the slimmer, I have produced a cassette tape. It acts to reinforce your motivation and to give you further supportive and sympathetic insights into your real motives and attitudes. In addition, it contains another powerful method to improve your ability to visualise success in order to produce success.

It is available from the above addresses.

THE MIND & BODY DIET™

Dieting and your Doctor

DIETING AND YOUR DOCTOR

You should consult your doctor before starting any diet. Your doctor will be interested in the following information, which applies to all Uni-Vite products, i.e. all provide complete nutri- tion. Protein and carbohydrate levels vary between products, but the Personalised Diet Programme ensures that protein and calorie minima are met or exceeded.

Vitamin/Mineral profile

Nutrient	*Per serving*	*Per day (3 servings)*	*% RDA per day*	
Sodium	500mg	1500mg	At least 100%	(3)
Potassium	670mg	2010mg	At least 100%	(3)
Chloride	600mg	1800mg	At least 100%	(3)
Magnesium	116.7mg	350mg	At least 100%	(3)
Calcium	300mg	900mg	180%	(1,2,4)
Phosphorus	266.7mg	800mg	At least 100%	(3)
Iron	6.7mg	20mg	167%	(2,4)
Zinc	6.7mg	20mg	At least 100%	(3)
Copper	0.7mg	2mg	At least 100%	(3)
Manganese	1.0mg	2.9mg	At least 100%	(3)
Iodine	50µg	150µg	107%	(4)
Molybdenum	53.3µg	160µg	At least 100%	(3)
Chromium	20µg	60µg	At least 100%	(3)
Selenium	20µg	60µg	At least 100%	(3)
Vitamin A	0.3mg	1mg	133%	(1,2.4)
Vitamin D	1.0µg	3µg	120%	(4)
Vitamin E	3.3mg	10mg	At least 100%	(3)
Vitamin C	23.3mg	70mg	233%	(1,2,4)
Vitamin K	23.3µg	70µg	At least 100%	(3)
Pantothenic Acid	2.3mg	7mg	At least 100%	(3)
Thiamin (Vitamin B_1)	0.7mg	2mg	167%	(4)
Riboflavin (Vitamin B_2)	0.7mg	2mg	125%	(1,4)
Niacin	6.3mg	19mg	106%	(1,4)
Pyridoxine (Vitamin B_6)	1mg	3mg	At least 100%	(3)

Folic Acid	133μg	400μg	133%	(1,2,4
Biotin	66μg	200μg	At least 100%	(3)
Vitamin B12	1.0μg	3μg	150%	(4)
Choline	75mg	225mg	*	
Inositol	20mg	60mg	*	

RDA – Recommended Daily Allowance

(1) DHSS Recommended Daily Amounts 1981 (for men)

(2) DHSS Recommended Daily Amounts 1981 (for women)

(3) National Academy of Science RDA (revised 1980)

(4) Recommendation of Food Labelling Regulations 1984

* No minimum amounts established

A graphic representation of how the calorie deficit is achieved on a Uni-Vite diet

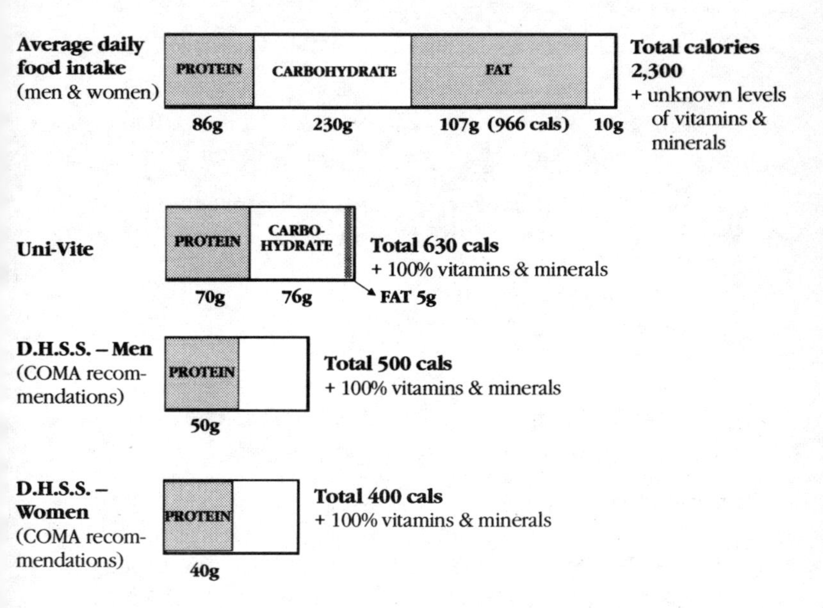

Notes

1. The calorie deficit on the Uni-Vite diet is achieved by virtually eliminating fat and reducing carbohydrate, whilst maintaining protein and actually increasing vitamin and minerals levels.

2. The Uni-Vite Gold diet above is an example of a typical personalised diet using Uni-Vite products.

Classification

The Uni-Vite Personalised Diet Programme can be classified as a Low Calorie Diet. These have been described in the most comprehensive survey as "the most important recent development in the treatment of obesity" – American College of Physicians (Wadden et al 1983). It is **not** a Very Low Calorie Diet as defined by C.O.M.A. in its report "The use of Very Low Calorie Diets in

Obesity", as it is—except in specific circumstances where full medical supervision is available—in excess of 600 calories per day total intake.

Effective

The *average* weight loss with LCD's is 20 kgs (44lbs) when treatments have a minimum 12 week duration (Wadden 1983).

In contrast only 10% of patients treated with conventional therapies ever achieve a weight loss of 20 kg (Asher and Dietz 1972)

Safety

The Uni-Vite Personalised Diet Programme contains the full level of protein as recommended by the World Health Organisation and by the DHSS in the C.O.M.A. Report.

This is important, as not only have over 3 million people safely used the Uni-Vite Diet Programme but the Wadden Survey (1983) concluded "evidence of safety is provided by the results of 24-hour Holter monitoring. Cardiac performance is not adversely affected by formula diets of high quality protein—in fact it may actually be improved."

Blood pressure

Weight loss in obese hypertensives is very often accompanied by a reduction in blood pressure. This takes place after as little as one week for most patients, and in one study over 65% of hypertensive patients achieved a normotensive state at the successful conclusion of the Low Calorie Diet regime. Patients on diuretic agents may no longer require them. Kirschener (1988) reported blood pressure was normalised in 71% of obese hypertensives after following a low-calorie diet.

Hyperlipidaemia

Significant reductions in serum cholesterol and triglyceride levels usually accompany weight loss on a Low Calorie Diet (Schouten et al 1981). Hypertriglyceridaemia was normalised in 77% and lowered, but not to normal, in 23% of obese hypertriglyceridaemic patients after weight loss (Kirshener 1988).

Diabetes

Low Calorie Diets have been shown to be effective in the treatment of obese type II diabetics (Genuth 1979). Patients may tolerate withdrawal from hypoglycaemia agents or reduction in insulin dose. Kirshener (1988) found all patients on oral drugs could discontinue therapy. Insulin was discontinued in 87% of cases and insulin dose decreased for 10% of patients.

Side effects

Side effects are not common, but in a small number of patients the concentration of the nutrients in the product may bring about short term postural hypotension, diarrhoea, or halitosis. In most cases these can be alleviated, or at least reduced, by drinking 4–6 pints (2–3 litres) of fluid in addition to the diet.

Non complications

Kirshener (1988) reported coronary by-pass surgery (8 patients), major breast surgery (12 patients) and pregnancies (6 patients) occurring while patients were on a low-calorie diet. All were without problems. The low-calorie diet was discontinued when the pregnancies were diagnosed.

Routine monitoring

Regular clinical examinations and monitoring of serum, uric acid, potassium, ECG, haemoglobin and liver enzymes (alanine and aspartate transaminase) are recommended in patients losing more than 14kg (30lbs).

Clinical trials

Clinical trials on the Uni-Vite diet have been conducted at the University of Surrey, the University of Barcelona, the Teutoburgerwald Clinic, West Germany, the University of Otago, New Zealand, and the University of Utrecht. They cover non-obese as well as obese subjects.

The weight loss over a 30 day period at calorie levels varying from 400–600 was consistent at an average 16 lbs (7.3 kg).

Contraindications

The use of low-calorie formula diets is not recommended in the case of:

Recent stroke or major heart attack
Type 1 diabetes
Gilbert's disease
Pregnancy and lactation
Steroid therapy
Children under 15

Special categories of dieters

Special Category	*Suitable Varieties*
Vegetarian	All Products
Gluten free	All Micro Drinks Uni-Vite Gold: Vanilla and Chocolate Whole Meals: Chilli
Patients taking mono-amine oxidase inhibitors	Micro Drinks: Banana, Butterscotch, Coffee, Strawberry and Vanilla Micro Soups: Vegetable Uni-Vite Gold: Vanilla & Vegetable Whole Meals: Chilli and Curry
Lactose intolerance	All Micro Bars and Whole Meals

Directions for use on pack

Each carton of Uni-Vite Diet product contains the following warning:

IMPORTANT NOTICE FOR YOUR SLIMMING SAFETY

You should consult your doctor before starting this or any other diet. Individuals who have conditions such as heart or cardiovascular disease, stroke, kidney disease, diabetes, gout, chronic infections or hypoglycaemia should diet only under medical supervision. Pregant women and nursing mothers (or even women planning to start a family) should not be put on any weight loss programme without their doctor's approval. Only use a Uni-Vite Personalised Diet as your sole source of nutrition for up to three consecutive weeks at any one time if it is below 600 calories, and only if you are dieting under your doctor's supervision.

The plateau phase

Some dieters find that, after a period of weight loss, their weight stabilises before they have reached their target. This is what is known as the "plateau phase" and it is due to one of the following reasons:

1. On commencing a weight loss diet, the glycogen stored is used. Each gramme of glycogen is associated with 4g of water, so when the carbohydrate is mobilised the water is lost. Hence the diuresis in the first week. However, in subsequent weeks the glycogen stores begin to build up again and water is retained with it. Therefore, it may seem that a large amount of weight is lost in the first week, but nothing is lost in the next few weeks. Nevertheless, fat is being lost, and it is only the fluctuations in fluid balance which are hiding the fat loss.
2. Fluid retention may also occur pre-menstrually in women and may mask loss of adipose tissue. However, since a pound of fat occupies a larger volume than a pound of water, if the dieter measures her waist and hip circumference she can note a volume decrease, even though it is not registered on the scales.

General substantiation

Wadden, Stunkard & Brownell – The most comprehensive survey of Low Calorie Diet studies was undertaken in 1983 by Wadden, Stunkard and Brownell.

They surveyed controlled studies covering a total of 1687 dieters and concluded: "Large, rapid weight losses and reduction in risk factors make the use of low-calorie diets attractive."

"Thus a comprehensive program combining low-calorie diets (to achieve a large initial weight loss) with nutrition education, exercise, training and behaviour modification would appear to be the next step."

Uni-Vite Nutrition has produced just such a comprehensive programme.

Van Gaal – A six week treatment with a 500 calorie formula diet containing 60g of protein, showed an average weight loss of 14.4kg, but lean body mass remained unchanged.

Apfelbaum – Has found that, after a low calorie (560 cal) diet containing 55g of protein, relatively obese young women will maintain their lean body mass intact and that no incident has been reported on such a diet in a series of 4000 outpatients over 13 years.

A further study on moderately overweight ambulatory patients, using a 560 calorie diet with 70g of protein, showed nitrogen equilibrium reached on the eighth day—i.e. no loss of lean body mass. Adequate potassium 2g a day together with 100% RDAs of vitamins and minerals were important.

THE UNI-VITE MICRO DIET USER STUDY

In March/April 1985 a study was conducted at the University of Surrey to examine the experiences of Uni-Vite Diet users.

855 users responded to the survey. Below is a summary of the result.

Weight loss

95% had tried to lose weight before.
94% found it easier with Uni-Vite's Diet

Lay Support

77% said the role of the Advisor was important in achieving their weight loss.

Doctors' Attitude

71% of doctors, when asked, actively encouraged the use the Uni-Vite Diet.

Health Aspects

89% felt well on the Uni-Vite Diet. 71% noticed a specific improvement in their health.

Weight Maintenance

87% found it easier to maintain their weight with the Uni-Vite Diet.
50%+ had kept the weight off for up to one year.
89% used the Uni-Vite Diet to help maintain their weight.

Eating Habits

80% reported changes in eating habits since using the Uni-Vite Diet.

The changes reported included:

Reduced consumption of:	*Increased consumption of:*
Butter and margarine	Green vegetables
Meat	Fruit
Biscuits	Fish
Sweets	Wholemeal bread
Puddings	
Fried food	
Nuts	
Crisps	

N.B. All the evidence is that dietary advice as a strategy to **lose** weight is good in theory but relatively ineffective in practice. When slimmers have already lost weight, they are then more willing to modify habits. The Uni-Vite Programme recognises this reality.

SOME KEY POINTS ON THE PSYCHOLOGY OF SLIMMING

1. The importance of the competitive element

One of the most influential researchers in the field is Dr Kelly Brownell, Professor of Psychiatry at the University of Pennsylvania. Citing motivation as a key factor in success, he has reported on several competitive programmes, e.g. teams within a manufacturing plant or teams from individual corporations, banks, insurance companies, etc. In contrast to worksite education programmes without a competitive element, where drop-out rate ran at 50% and weight losses were small, the addition of a competition/reward element reduced drop-out to 5% and produced good average weight losses.

2 Differentiating between lapse and relapse

Brownell has convincingly put the case for inviting slimmers to draw the distinction between a lapse and a relapse. Acknowledging work from researchers Prochaska and Di Clemente, he suggests that lapses are commonly associated with social and situational factors—whereas relapses occur during negative emotional states. This leads to the clear need to assist in avoiding high risk situations to prevent the original relapse but, if it should occur, to encourage a positive emotional response, e.g. treat the situation as a learning occasion. Hence the emphasis on coping skills in the Mind & Body Diet Programme.

3. Response to treatment

a. As might be expected, early and significant initial weight losses definitely tend to predict long-term success. So does a programme involving self-reported compliance, i.e. use of the "feedback chart".

b. More interestingly, patients who struggle to a moderate degree to adhere to a diet programme appear to do well later—presumably because they have, indeed, learned coping skills.

c. One of the most important coping skills seems to be a strong urge to act quickly if a personal weight re-gain of, say, 3 lbs is experienced.

4. Characteristics of the obese

We have not found consistent specific traits that characterise overweight v. normal weight people. There are, however, indications that obese people who offer most resistance to treatment do share certain characteristics.

Kreitler, writing in the International Journal of Obesity 1988, summarises key cognitive factors as being:

* Unwillingness to accept limits on behaviour
* Low self-control
* Unwillingness to express hostility
* Unwillingness to express emotions
* Self-identity not very strong
* External orientation

5. Group motivation

Brownell, '84, Miller, '81, and Wilson, '85, have all found that support from friends (and family) is strongly correlated with long-term success.

Conversely, stressful inter-personal relationships appear to be involved in almost 50% of relapse situations.

The practical use of small self-help groups is well documented for a variety of purposes from dieting to alcohol abuse.

Professor John Flowers, an expert on group dynamics, has shown that the most effective way to change attitudes is neither individual nor large group therapy, but small groups of between 6 and 12 people.

Furthermore, his experience indicates that certain types of people find particular strength from small groups.

These include people who:

* benefit from additional emotional support outside their family
* are insightful and enjoy exploring issues
* are happy to take responsibility for their own progress
* plateau during the diet phase.

Important is the freedom that members develop to express fears and then to begin to work out solutions—solutions that often benefit everyone. Uni-Vite has found that many of the attitudes and coping skills that a group develops during "Team Trim" sessions extend to the other areas of their lives, with great benefit.

Successful use of lay groups

Uni-Vite has, as mentioned in the "Mind & Body Diet", evolved a structured group support system called "Team Trimming".

A trained, but lay, leader facilitates a series of six group meetings. Input is by audio cassette plus a manual for each member based on this book.

Weight loss is taking place throughout the six week period and, since this is recommended to be via a low-calorie (approx. 600) formula diet, the weight loss is normally very encouraging.

There is a prize at the end for each successful member. All teams are given an identity and can enter for a significant monthly cash prize draw.

A high degree of enjoyment, motivation and success is achieved, and significant counselling skills can be developed by "Team Trim" leaders.

The aim is to help a group member acquire the necessary knowledge and skill for long-term weight maintenance in a supportive and friendly environment.

REFERENCES

1. Apfelbaum, M., Baights, F., Gaichetti, I., and Serog, P., *Effects of a high protein very-low-energy diet on ambulatory subjects with special reference to nitrogen balance,* 1981, International Journal of Obesity, 5, 117-130.

2. Asher, W.L. and Deitz, R.E., *Effectiveness of Weight Reduction involving "diet pills",* 1972, Current Therapeutic Research, 14, 510-524.

3. Bander, R., and Grindler, J., *Frogs into princes: Real people,* 1979, Press U.S.A.

4. Brownell, K. and Jeffery, R., *Improving long term weight loss: Pushing the limits of treatment,* 1987, Behaviour Therapy, 18, 353-374.

5. Brownell, K., *Modern methods for weight control: The physiology and psychology of dieting,* 1987, 12, p122.

6. Brownell, K., *Understanding and preventing relapse,* 1986, American Psychologist, 41, 719-765.

7. Brownell, K., *Weight loss competitions at the worksite: Impact on weight, morale and cost effectiveness,* 1984, Journal of Public Health, 74, 1283-1285.

8. DHSS, Report on Health and Social Subjects, *Recommended Daily Amounts of Food Energy and Nutrients for Groups of People in the United Kingdom,* Report by the Committee on Medical Aspects of Policy, Her Majesty's Stationery Office, London.

9. DHSS, Report on Health and Social Subjects, *The Use of Very Low Calorie Diets in Obesity,* Report by the Working Group on Very Low Calorie Diets of the Committee on Medical Aspects of Food Policy, Her Majesty's Stationery Office, London.

10. Genuth, S.M,. Vertes, V., and Hazelton, I., *Supplemental Fasting in the Treatment of Obesity,* l978, Recent Advances in Obesity Research 2, ed. Bray, G.A. 370-378, Newman, London.

11. Grimso, A., *Short and long term effect of lay groups on weight reduction,* 1981, British Medical Journal, 283, 1093-1095.

12. James, W.P.T., *Treatment of obesity: The constraints on success,* 1984, Clinics in Endocrinology and Metabolism, 13, 635-659.

13. Kreitler, S., Chemerinski, A., *The cognitive orientation of obesity,* 1988, International Journal of Obesity, 12, 403-405.

14. Kirschener, M.A., Schneider, G., Ertel, N.H., Gorman, J., *An eight year experience of a Very Low Calorie Formula Diet for the contr of major obesity,* 1988, International Journal of Obesity, 12, 69-80

15. Mahoney, M.J., *Self reward and self monitoring techniques for weight control,* 1974, Behaviour Therapy, 5, 48-57.

16. Miller, P.M., and Sims, K.L., *Evaluation and component analysis a comprehensive weight control program,* 1981, International Jou of Obesity, 5, 57-66.

17. Peri, M.G., et al, *Maintenance strategies for the treatment of obesity,* 1984, Journal of Consulting and Clinical Psychology, 52, 404-413.

18. Schouten, J.A., et al. *The influence of low calorie protein-carbohydrate diets on serum lipids in obese subjects,* 1981, Internationa Journal of Obesity, 5, 333-339

19. Stunkard, A.J., *Behaviour modification in the treatment of obesit* 1979, Archives of General Psychiatry, 36, 801-806.

20. Tuck, M.L., Sowers, J.Dornfeld, L., Kledzik, G., Maxwell, M., *The effect of weight reduction on blood pressure, plasma renin activi and plasma aldosterone levels in obese patients,* 1981, New Engla Journal of Medicine, 304, 903-933.

21. Van Gaal, L.F., Snyders, D., De Leeuw, I.H., Bekaert, J.L., *Anthropometric and calorimetric evidence for the protein sparing effect of a new protein supplemented low calorie preparation,* 1985, American Journal of Clinical Nutrition, 41, 540-544.

22. Wadden, T.A., Stunkard, A.J., Brownell, K.D., *Very Low Calorie Diets: Their Efficacy, Safety and Future,* 1983 Annals of Internal Medicine, 99, 675-684.

23. Wilson, G.T., *Psychological prognostic factors in the treatment of obesity,* Recent Advances in Obesity Research, 1985, 4, 301-311.

24. Wing, R.R., Jeffrey, R.W., *Outpatient treatments of obesity: a comparison of methodology and clinical results,* 1979, International Journal of Obesity, 3, 261-272.

25 Wynn, V., Abraham, R.R., Densem, J.W., *Method for estimating rate of fat loss during treatment of obesity by calorie restriction,* 1985, The Lancet, 1, 482-486.

Uni-Vite is marketed in: Australia, Bahamas, Canada, Eire, France, Holland, Hong Kong, Iceland, Israel, Japan, Malaysia, Malta, Nigeria, New Zealand, Oman, Pakistan, Portugal, Spain, Sweden, Trinidad, U.S.A and West Germany.

NOTES

NOTES

NOTES

NOTES

NOTES

NOTES

NOTES

NOTES

NOTES

NOTES

NOTES

NOTES

NOTES